Excel for Statistics

Excel for Statistics is a series of textbooks that explain how to use Excel to solve statistics problems in various fields of study. Professors, students, and practitioners will find these books teach how to make Excel work best in their respective field. Applications include any discipline that uses data and can benefit from the power and simplicity of Excel. Books cover all the steps for running statistical analyses in Excel 2016, Excel 2013, Excel 2010 and Excel 2007. The approach also teaches critical statistics skills, making the books particularly applicable for statistics courses taught outside of mathematics or statistics departments.

Series editor: Thomas J. Quirk

The following books are in this series:

T.J. Quirk, S. Cummings, *Excel 2016 for Social Work Statistics*, Excel for Statistics. Springer International Publishing AG 2017.

T.J. Quirk, E. Rhiney, *Excel 2016 for Marketing Statistics: A Guide to Solving Practical Problems*, Excel for Statistics. Springer International Publishing Switzerland 2016.

T.J. Quirk, *Excel 2016 for Engineering Statistics: A Guide to Solving Practical Problems*, Excel for Statistics. Springer International Publishing Switzerland 2016.

T.J. Quirk, *Excel 2016 for Business Statistics: A Guide to Solving Practical Problems*, Excel for Statistics. Springer International Publishing Switzerland 2016.

T.J. Quirk, M. Quirk, H.F. Horton, *Excel 2016 for Biological and Life Sciences Statistics: A Guide to Solving Practical Problems*, Excel for Statistics. Springer International Publishing 2016.

T.J. Quirk, M. Quirk, H.F. Horton, *Excel 2016 for Physical Sciences Statistics: A Guide to Solving Practical Problems*, Excel for Statistics. Springer International Publishing 2016.

T.J. Quirk. *Excel 2016 for Educational and Psychological Statistics: A Guide to Solving Practical Problems*, Excel for Statistics. Springer International Publishing Switzerland 2016.

T.J. Quirk, *Excel 2016 for Social Science Statistics: A Guide to Solving Practical Problems*, Excel for Statistics. Springer International Publishing Switzerland 2016.

T.J. Quirk, S. Cummings, *Excel 2016 for Health Services Management Statistics: A Guide to Solving Practical Problems*. Excel for Statistics. Springer International Publishing Switzerland 2016.

T.J. Quirk, J. Palmer-Schuyler, *Excel 2016 for Human Resource Management Statistics: A Guide to Solving Practical Problems*, Excel for Statistics. Springer International Publishing Switzerland 2016.

T.J. Quirk, M. Quirk, H.F. Horton. *Excel 2016 for Environmental Sciences Statistics: A Guide to Solving Practical Problems*, Excel for Statistics. Springer International Publishing Switzerland 2016.

T.J. Quirk, J. Palmer-Schuyler, *Excel 2013 for Human Resource Management Statistics: A Guide to Solving Practical Problems*, Excel for Statistics. Springer International Publishing Switzerland 2016.

T.J. Quirk, S. Cummings, *Excel 2013 for Health Services Management Statistics: A Guide to Solving Practical Problems*. Excel for Statistics. Springer International Publishing Switzerland 2016.

T.J. Quirk, M. Quirk, H.F. Horton, *Excel 2013 for Physical Sciences Statistics: A Guide to Solving Practical Problems*. Excel for Statistics. Springer International Publishing Switzerland 2016.

T.J. Quirk. *Excel 2013 for Educational and Psychological Statistics: A Guide to Solving Practical Problems*, Excel for Statistics. Springer International Publishing Switzerland 2015.

T.J. Quirk, M. Quirk, H.F. Horton, *Excel 2013 for Biological and Life Sciences Statistics: A Guide to Solving Practical Problems*, Excel for Statistics. Springer International Publishing 2015.

T.J. Quirk, *Excel 2013 for Social Science Statistics: A Guide to Solving Practical Problems*, Excel for Statistics. Springer International Publishing Switzerland 2015.

T.J. Quirk, *Excel 2013 for Business Statistics: A Guide to Solving Practical Problems*, Excel for Statistics. Springer International Publishing Switzerland 2015.

T.J. Quirk, *Excel 2013 for Engineering Statistics: A Guide to Solving Practical Problems*. Excel for Statistics. Springer International Publishing Switzerland 2015.

T.J. Quirk, M. Quirk, H.F. Horton, *Excel 2013 for Environmental Sciences Statistics: A Guide to Solving Practical Problems*. Excel for Statistics. Springer International Publishing Switzerland 2015.

Additional Statistics books by Dr. Tom Quirk that have been published by Springer

T.J. Quirk, *Excel 2010 for Engineering Statistics: A Guide to Solving Practical Problems*. Springer International Publishing Switzerland 2014.

T.J. Quirk, S. Cummings, *Excel 2010 for Health Services Management Statistics: A Guide to Solving Practical Problems*. Springer International Publishing Switzerland 2014.

T.J. Quirk, M. Quirk, H. Horton, *Excel 2010 for Physical Sciences Statistics: A Guide to Solving Practical Problems*. Springer International Publishing Switzerland 2013.

T.J. Quirk, M. Quirk, H.F. Horton, *Excel 2010 for Biological and Life Sciences Statistics: A Guide to Solving Practical Problems*. Springer Science+Business Media New York 2013.

T.J. Quirk, M. Quirk, H.F. Horton, *Excel 2007 for Biological and Life Sciences Statistics: A Guide to Solving Practical Problems*. Springer Science+Business Media New York 2013.

T.J. Quirk, *Excel 2010 for Social Science Statistics: A Guide to Solving Practical Problems*. Springer Science+Business Media New York 2012.

T.J. Quirk, Excel 2010 for *Educational and Psychological Statistics: A Guide to Solving Practical Problems*. Springer Science+Business Media New York 2012.

T.J. Quirk, *Excel 2007 for Business Statistics: A Guide to Solving Practical Problems*. Springer Science+Business Media New York 2012.

T.J. Quirk, *Excel 2007 for Social Science Statistics: A Guide to Solving Practical Problems*. Springer Science+Business Media New York 2012.

T.J. Quirk, *Excel 2007 for Educational and Psychological Statistics: A Guide to Solving Practical Problems*. Springer Science+Business Media New York 2012.

More information about this series at http://www.springer.com/series/13491

Thomas J. Quirk • Simone Cummings

Excel 2016 for Social Work Statistics

A Guide to Solving Practical Problems

Springer

Thomas J. Quirk
Webster University
St. Louis, MO, USA

Simone Cummings
Webster University
St. Louis, MO, USA

Excel for Statistics
ISBN 978-3-319-66220-6 ISBN 978-3-319-66221-3 (eBook)
DOI 10.1007/978-3-319-66221-3

Library of Congress Control Number: 2017951017

This Springer imprint is published by Springer Nature
The registered company is Springer International Publishing AG
The registered company address is: Gewerbestrasse 11, 6330 Cham, Switzerland

This book is dedicated to the more than 3,000 students I have taught at Webster University's campuses in St. Louis, London, and Vienna; the students at Principia College in Elsah, Illinois; and the students at the Cooperative State University of Baden-Wuerttemberg in Heidenheim, Germany. These students taught me a great deal about the art of teaching. I salute them all, and I thank them for helping me to become a better teacher.

Thomas J. Quirk

To Don, my husband and best friend; to our children, Nina and Madison; and to my parents, Albert and Wava. Thank you.

Simone Cummings

Preface

Excel 2016 for Social Work Statistics: A Guide to Solving Practical Problems is intended for anyone looking to learn the basics of applying Excel's powerful statistical tools to their social work courses or work activities. If understanding statistics isn't your strongest suit, you are not especially mathematically inclined, or if you are wary of computers, then this is the right book for you.

Here you'll learn how to use key statistical tests using Excel without being overpowered by the underlying statistical theory. This book clearly and methodically shows and explains how to create and use these statistical tests to solve practical problems in social work.

Excel is an easily available computer program for students, instructors, and managers. It is also an effective teaching and learning tool for quantitative analyses in social work courses. The powerful numerical computational ability and the graphical functions available in Excel make learning statistics much easier than in years past. However, this is the first book to show Excel's capabilities to more effectively teach social work statistics; it also focuses exclusively on this topic in an effort to render the subject matter not only applicable and practical but also easy to comprehend and apply.

Unique features of this book:

- You will be told each step of the way, not only *how* to use Excel but also *why* you are doing each step so that you can understand what you are doing, and not merely learn how to use statistical tests by rote.
- Includes specific objectives embedded in the text for each concept, so you can know the purpose of the Excel steps.
- Includes 163 color screenshots so that you can be sure you are performing the Excel steps correctly.
- This book is a tool that can be used either by itself or along with *any* good statistics book.
- Practical examples and problems are taken from social work.

- Statistical theory and formulas are explained in clear language without bogging you down in mathematical fine points.
- You will learn both how to write statistical formulas using Excel and how to use Excel's drop-down menus that will create the formulas for you.
- This book does not come with a CD of Excel files which you can upload to your computer. Instead, you'll be shown how to create each Excel file yourself. In a work situation, your colleagues will not give you an Excel file; you will be expected to create your own. This book will give you ample practice in developing this important skill.
- Each chapter presents the steps needed to solve a practical social work problem using Excel. In addition, there are three practice problems at the end of each chapter so you can test your new knowledge of statistics. The answers to these problems appear in Appendix A.
- A "Practice Test" is given in Appendix B to test your knowledge at the end of the book. The answers to these practical social work problems appear in Appendix C.

This book is appropriate for use in any course in social work statistics (at both undergraduate and graduate levels) as well as for managers who want to improve the usefulness of their Excel skills.

Dr. Tom Quirk, a current Professor of Marketing at the George Herbert Walker School of Business & Technology at Webster University in St. Louis, Missouri (USA), teaches Marketing Statistics, Marketing Research, and Pricing Strategies. At the beginning of his academic career, Prof. Quirk spent six years in educational research at the American Institutes for Research and Educational Testing Service. He then taught Social Psychology, Educational Psychology, and General Psychology at Principia College in Elsah, Illinois (USA). He has published articles in the *Journal of Educational Psychology, Journal of Educational Research, Review of Educational Research, Journal of Educational Measurement, Educational Technology, The Elementary School Journal, Journal of Secondary Education, Educational Horizons, and Phi Delta Kappan*. Professor Quirk has published more than 20 articles in professional journals and presented more than 20 papers at professional meetings, including annual meetings of the American Educational Research Association, the American Psychological Association, and the National Council on Measurement in Education. He holds a B.S. in Mathematics from John Carroll University, both an M.A. in Education and a Ph.D. in Educational Psychology from Stanford University, and an M.B.A. from the University of Missouri-St. Louis.

Prof. Simone Cummings is currently Dean of the Walker School of Business and Technology at Webster University in St. Louis, Missouri, USA, where she also teaches Statistics for Health Administration, Healthcare Finance, and Introduction to Healthcare Services. She holds both a B.S.B.A. and an M.H.A from Washington University in St. Louis and a Ph.D. in Health Management and Policy from the University of North Carolina at Chapel Hill. Prof. Cummings has served on the Board of the Association of University Programs in Health Administration and currently serves as a Fellow for the Commission on Accreditation of Healthcare

Management Education. She has experience consulting and working in a variety of healthcare delivery organizations, including hospitals, clinics, and physician groups. She has conducted clinical and health services research for more than ten years and published articles in *Health Services Research, Healthcare Executive, Trustee, Academic Emergency Medicine, Journal of National Medical Association, and Academic Medicine.*

St. Louis, MO

Thomas J. Quirk
Simone M. Cummings

Acknowledgements

Excel 2016 for Social Work Statistics: A Guide to Solving Practical Problems is the result of inspiration from three important people: my two daughters and my wife. Jennifer Quirk McLaughlin invited me to visit her MBA classes several times at the University of the Witwatersrand in Johannesburg, South Africa. These visits to a first-rate MBA program convinced me there was a need for a book to teach students how to solve practical problems using Excel. Meghan Quirk-Horton's dogged dedication to learning the many statistical techniques needed to complete her PhD dissertation illustrated the need for a statistics book that would make this daunting task more user-friendly. And Lynne Buckley-Quirk was the number-one cheerleader for this project from the beginning, always encouraging me and helping me remain dedicated to completing it.

Michael Penn, our editor at Springer, shepherded this book through the idea stages until it reached its final form. His encouragement and support were vital to this book seeing the light of day. We thank him for being such an outstanding product champion throughout this process.

Thomas J. Quirk

Special thanks to my coauthor, Tom Quirk, for inviting me to work with him on this project and for his wonderful collaboration. Special thanks also to our editor at Springer, Michael Penn, for his support and assistance.

Simone M. Cummings

Contents

Chapter 1
Sample Size, Mean, Standard Deviation, and Standard Error of the Mean

Social work attempts to improve people's quality of life toward their full potential as a person, as a group member, and in their community.

This chapter deals with how you can use Excel to find the average (i.e., "mean") of a set of scores, the standard deviation of these scores (STDEV), and the standard error of the mean (s.e.) of these scores. All three of these statistics are used frequently and form the basis for additional statistical tests.

1.1 Mean

The *mean* is the "arithmetic average" of a set of scores. When my daughter was in the fifth grade, she came home from school with a sad face and said that she didn't get "averages." The book she was using described how to find the mean of a set of scores, and so I said to her:

> "Jennifer, you add up all the scores and divide by the number of numbers that you have."
>
> She gave me "that look," and said: "Dad, this is serious!" She thought I was teasing her. So I said:
>
> "See these numbers in your book; add them up. What is the answer?" (She did that.)
>
> "Now, how many numbers do you have?" (She answered that question.)
>
> "Then, take the number you got when you added up the numbers, and divide that number by the number of numbers that you have."

She did that, and found the correct answer. You will use that same reasoning now, but it will be much easier for you because Excel will do all of the steps for you.

We will call this average of the scores the "mean" which we will symbolize as: $\bar{X}$, and we will pronounce it as: "Xbar."

The formula for finding the mean with your calculator looks like this:

$$\bar{X} = \frac{\sum X}{n} \tag{1.1}$$

T.J. Quirk, S. Cummings, *Excel 2016 for Social Work Statistics*, Excel for Statistics, DOI 10.1007/978-3-319-66221-3_1

The symbol Σ is the Greek letter sigma, which stands for "sum." It tells you to add up all the scores that are indicated by the letter X, and then to divide your answer by n (the number of numbers that you have).

Let's give a simple example:

Length of Stay (LOS) is the number of calendar days a patient stays in a health care facility from admission to discharge. Suppose that you had these six LOS scores for a random sample of mothers who gave birth and were discharged in the past two weeks:

6
4
5
3
2
5

To find the mean of these scores, you add them up, and then divide by the number of scores. So, the mean is: 25/6 = 4.17

1.2 Standard Deviation

The *standard deviation* tells you "how close the scores are to the mean." If the standard deviation is a small number, this tells you that the scores are "bunched together" close to the mean. If the standard deviation is a large number, this tells you that the scores are "spread out" a greater distance from the mean. The formula for the standard deviation (which we will call STDEV) and use the letter, S, to symbolize is:

$$\text{STDEV} = S = \sqrt{\frac{\sum (X - \bar{X})^2}{n - 1}} \tag{1.2}$$

The formula look complicated, but what it asks you to do is this:

1. Subtract the mean from each score $(X - \bar{X})$.
2. Then, square the resulting numbers to make each a positive number.
3. Then, add up these squared numbers to get a total score.
4. Then, take this total score and divide it by n − 1 (where n stands for the number of numbers that you have).
5. The final step is to take the square root of the number you found in step 4.

You will not be asked to compute the standard deviation using your calculator in this book, but you could see examples of how it is computed in any basic statistics book (e.g. Bowers 2008; Engel and Shutt 2013). Instead, we will use Excel to find the standard deviation of a set of scores. When we use Excel on the six numbers we gave in the description of the mean above, you will find that the *STDEV* of these numbers, S, is 1.47.

1.3 Standard Error of the Mean

The formula for the *standard error of the mean* (*s.e.*, which we will use $S_{\bar{X}}$ to symbolize) is:

$$\text{s.e.} = S_{\bar{X}} = \frac{S}{\sqrt{n}} \tag{1.3}$$

To find ***s.e.***, all you need to do is to take the standard deviation, STDEV, and divide it by the square root of n, where n stands for the "number of numbers" that you have in your data set. In the example under the standard deviation description above, the *s.e.* = 0.60. (You can check this on your calculator.)

If you want to learn more about the standard deviation and the standard error of the mean, see Polit (2010) and Schneider (2010).

Now, let's learn how to use Excel to find the sample size, the mean, the standard deviation, and the standard error or the mean using Length of Stay (LOS) for adult men in a health care facility for eight men who were discharged in the past week. The hypothetical data appear in Fig. 1.1.

Fig. 1.1 Worksheet Data for Length of Stay (Practical Example)

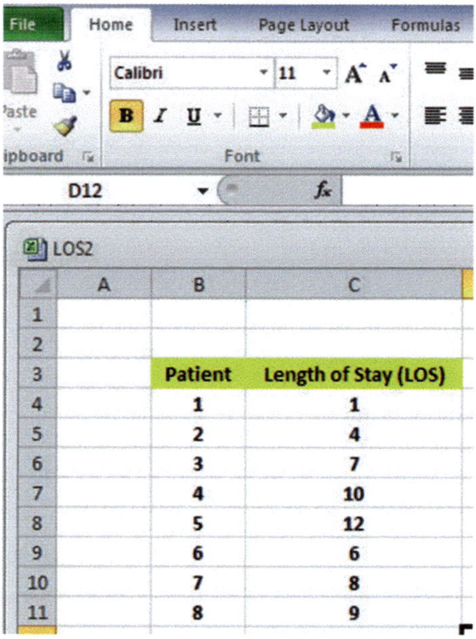

1.4 Sample Size, Mean, Standard Deviation, and Standard Error of the Mean

Objective:	To find the sample size (n), mean, standard deviation (STDEV), and standard error of the mean (s.e.) for these data

Start your computer, and click on the Excel 2016 icon to open a blank Excel spreadsheet.

Click on: Blank workbook

Enter the data in this way:

B3: Patient
C3: Length of Stay (LOS)
B4: 1

1.4.1 Using the Fill/Series/Columns Commands

Objective:	To add the sample numbers 2–8 in the patient column

Put pointer in B4
Home (top left of screen)

Important note: The "Paste" command should be on the top of your screen on the far left of the screen.

Important note: Notice the Excel commands at the top of your computer screen: ***File → Home → Insert → Page Layout → Formulas → etc.*** *If these commands ever "disappear" when you are using Excel, you need to click on "Home" at the top left of your screen to make them reappear!*

Fill (top right of screen: click on the Series down arrow; see Fig. 1.2)

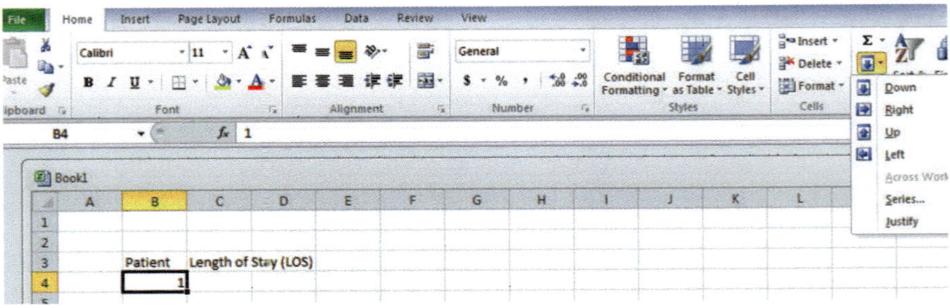

Fig. 1.2 Home/Fill/Series commands

Series
Columns
Step value: 1
Stop value: 8 (see Fig. 1.3)

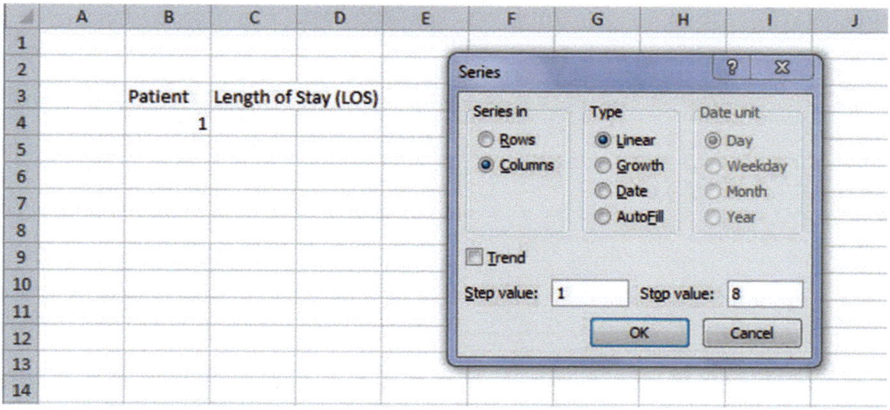

Fig. 1.3 Example of Dialogue Box for Fill/Series/Columns/Step Value/Stop Value commands

OK

The patient numbers should be identified as 1–8, with 8 in cell B11.

Now, enter the Length of Stay (LOS) figures in cells C4: C11. *(Note: Be sure to double-check your figures to make sure that they are correct or you will not get the correct answer!)*

Since your computer screen shows the information in a format that does not look professional, you need to learn how to "widen the column width" and how to "center the information" in a group of cells. Here is how you can do those two steps:

1.4.2 Changing the Width of a Column

Objective:	To make a column width wider so that all of the information fits inside that column

If you look at your computer screen, you can see that Column C is not wide enough so that all of the information fits inside this column. To make Column C wider:

Click on the letter, C, at the top of your computer screen
Place your mouse pointer on your computer at the far right corner of C until you create a "cross sign" on that corner

Left-click on your mouse, hold it down, and move this corner to the right until it is "wide enough to fit all of the data"
Take your finger off your mouse to set the new column width (see Fig. 1.4)

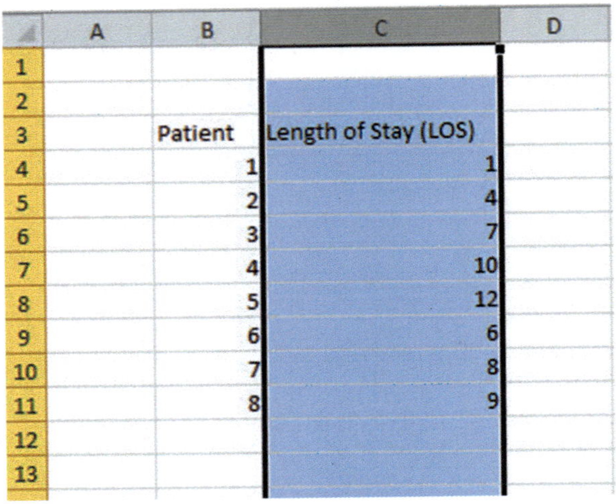

Fig. 1.4 Example of How to Widen the Column Width

Then, click on any empty cell (i.e., any blank cell) to "deselect" column C so that it is no longer a darker color on your screen.

When you widen a column, you will make all of the cells in all of the rows of this column that same width.

Now, let's go through the steps to center the information in both Column B and Column C.

1.4.3 Centering Information in a Range of Cells

Objective: To center the information in a group of cells

In order to make the information in the cells look "more professional," you can center the information using the following steps:
Left-click your mouse pointer on B3 and drag it to the right and down to highlight cells B3:C11 so that these cells appear in a darker color

At the top of your computer screen, you will see a set of "lines" in which all of the lines are "centered" to the same width under "Alignment" (it is the second icon at the bottom left of the Alignment box; see Fig. 1.5)

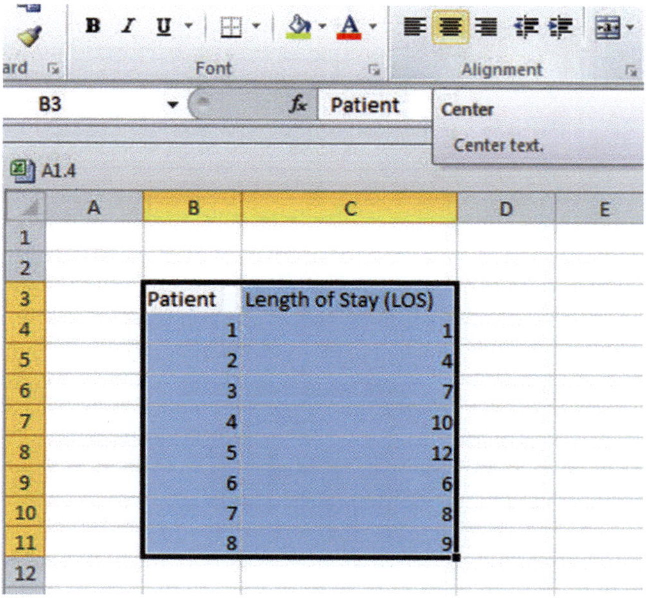

Fig. 1.5 Example of How to Center Information Within Cells

Click on this icon to center the information in the selected cells (see Fig. 1.6)

Fig. 1.6 Final Result of Centering Information in the Cells

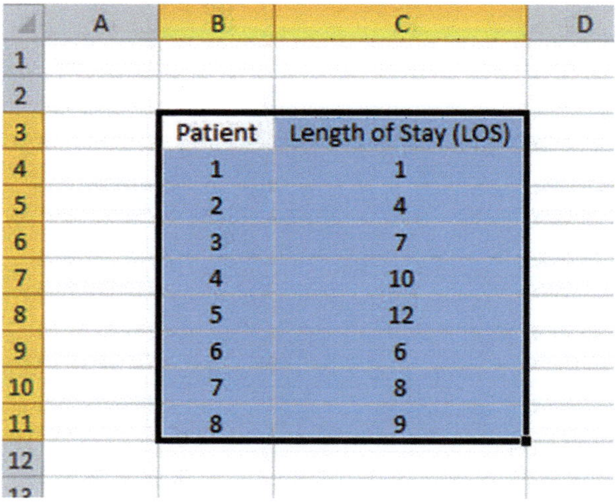

Since you will need to refer to the Length of Stay in your formulas, it will be much easier to do this if you "name the range of data" with a name instead of having to remember the exact cells (C4:C11) in which these figures are located. Let's call that group of cells: LOS, but we could give them any name that you want to use.

1.4.4 *Naming a Range of Cells*

Objective: To name the range of data for Length of Stay with the name: LOS

Highlight cells C4:C11 by left-clicking your mouse pointer on C4 and dragging it down to C11
Formulas (top left of your screen)
Define Name (top center of your screen)
LOS (type this name in the top box; see Fig. 1.7)

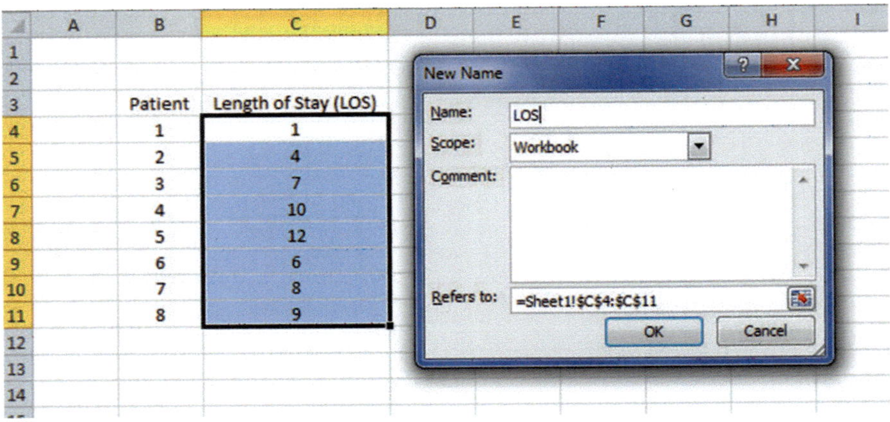

Fig. 1.7 Dialogue box for "naming a range of cells" with the name: LOS

OK
Then, click on any cell of your spreadsheet that does not have any information in it (i.e., it is an "empty cell") to deselect cells C4:C11
Now, add the following terms to your spreadsheet:

E6: n
E9: Mean
E12: STDEV
E15: s.e. (see Fig. 1.8)

Note: Whenever use a formula you must add an equal sign (=) at the beginning of the name of the function so that Excel knows that you indend to use a formula.

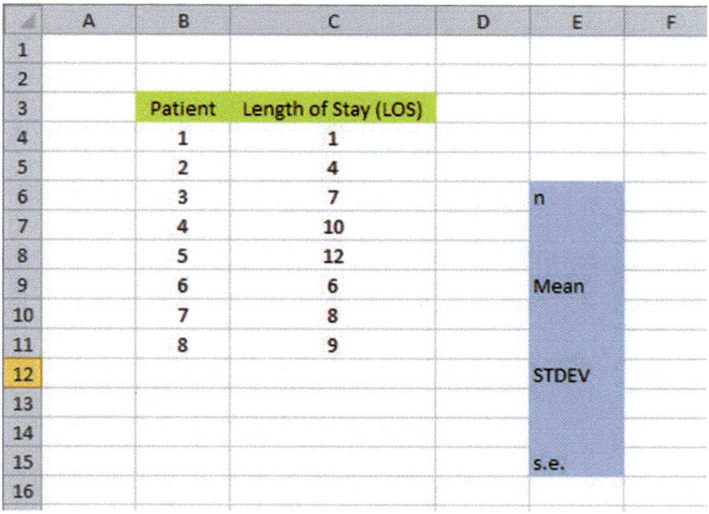

Fig. 1.8 Example of Entering the Sample Size, Mean, STDEV, and s.e. Labels

1.4.5 Finding the Sample Size Using the =COUNT Function

Objective:	To find the sample size (n) for these data using the =COUNT function

F6: =COUNT(LOS)

This command should insert the number 8 into cell F6 since there are eight patients in your sample.

1.4.6 Finding the Mean Score Using the =AVERAGE Function

Objective:	To find the mean LOS figure using the =AVERAGE function

F9: =AVERAGE(LOS)

This command should insert the number 7.125 into cell F9.

1.4.7 Finding the Standard Deviation Using the =STDEV Function

Objective:	To find the standard deviation (STDEV) using the =STDEV function

F12: =STDEV(LOS)

This command should insert the number 3.482097 into cell F12.

1.4.8 Finding the Standard Error of the Mean

Objective:	To find the standard error of the mean using a formula for these eight data points

F15: =F12/SQRT(8)

This command should insert the number 1.231107 into cell F15 (see Fig. 1.9).

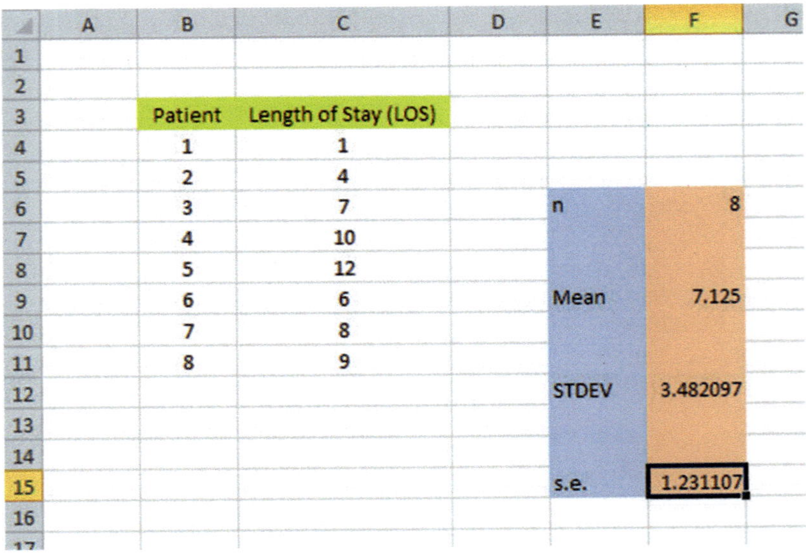

	A	B	C	D	E	F	G
1							
2							
3		Patient	Length of Stay (LOS)				
4		1	1				
5		2	4				
6		3	7		n	8	
7		4	10				
8		5	12				
9		6	6		Mean	7.125	
10		7	8				
11		8	9				
12					STDEV	3.482097	
13							
14							
15					s.e.	1.231107	
16							

Fig. 1.9 Example of Using Excel Formulas for Sample Size, Mean, STDEV, and s.e.

Important note: Throughout this book, be sure to double-check all of the figures in your spreadsheet to make sure that they are in the correct cells, or the formulas will not work correctly!

1.4.8.1 Formatting Numbers in Number Format (Two Decimal Places)

Objective: To convert the mean, STDEV, and s.e. to two decimal places

Highlight cells F9:F15

Home (top left of screen)

Look under "Number" at the top center of your screen. In the bottom right corner, gently place your mouse pointer on you screen at the bottom of the .00 .0 until it says: "Decrease Decimal" (see Fig. 1.10)

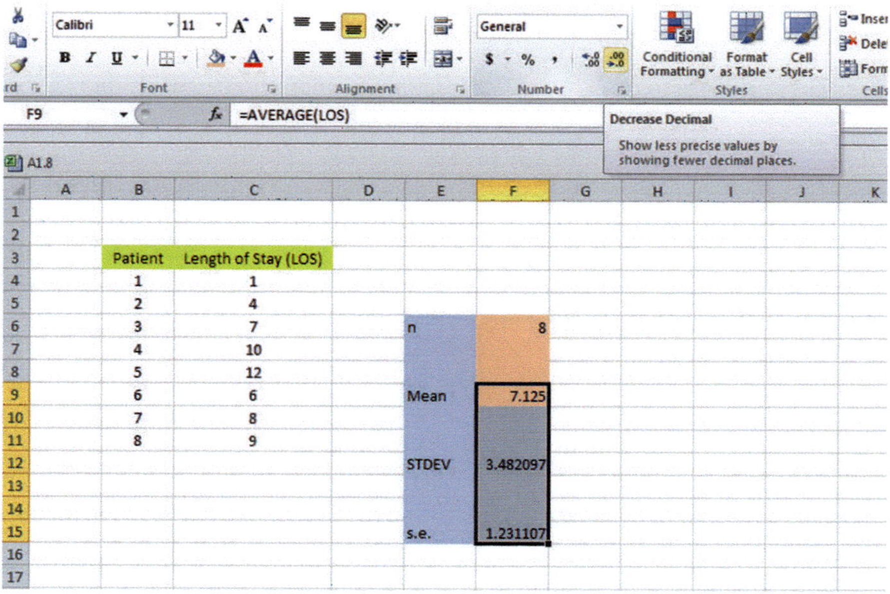

Fig. 1.10 Using the "Decrease Decimal Icon" to convert Numbers to Fewer Decimal Places

Click on this icon *once* and notice that the cells F9:F15 are now all in just two decimal places (see Fig. 1.11)

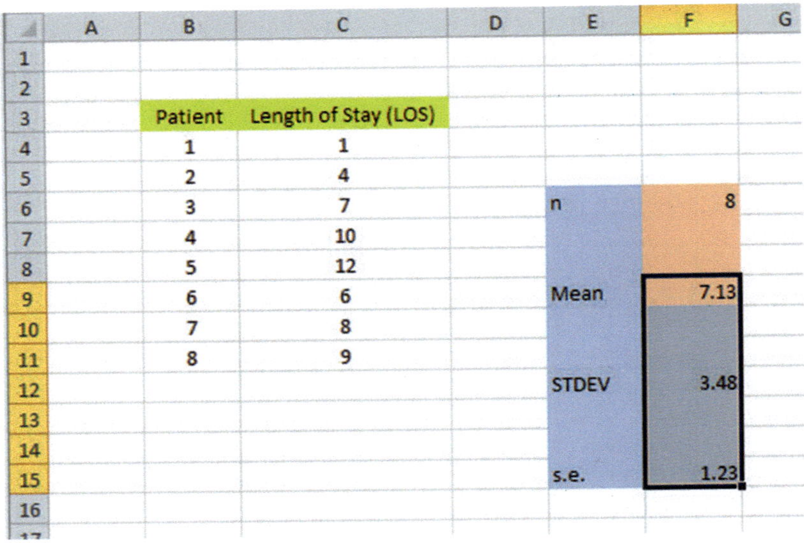

Fig. 1.11 Example of Converting Numbers to Two Decimal Places

Now, click on any "empty cell" on your spreadsheet to deselect cells F9:F15.

1.5 Saving a Spreadsheet

Objective: To save this spreadsheet with the name: LOS3

In order to save your spreadsheet so that you can retrieve it sometime in the future, your first decision is to decide "where" you want to save it. That is your decision and you have several choices. If it is your own computer, you can save it onto your hard drive (you need to ask someone how to do that on your computer). Or, you can save it onto a "CD" or onto a "flash drive." To save the spreadsheet, you need to complete these steps:

File
Save as

(select the place where you want to save the file by scrolling either down or up the bar on the left, and click on the place where you want to save the file; for example: This PC: My Documents location))

File name: LOS3 (enter this name to the right of File name; see Fig. 1.12)

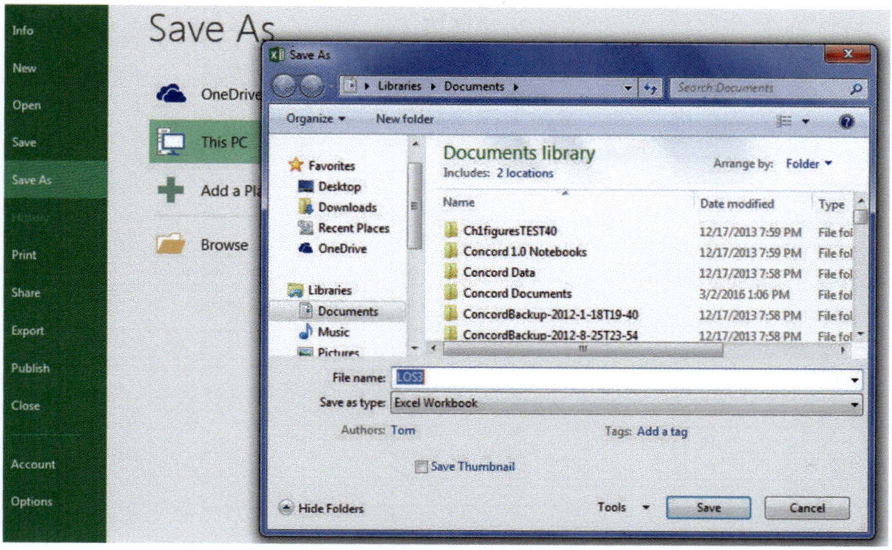

Fig. 1.12 Dialogue Box of Saving an Excel Workbook File as "LOS3" in My Documents location

Save

Important note: Be very careful to save your Excel file spreadsheet every few minutes so that you do not lose your information!

1.6 Printing a Spreadsheet

Objective: To print the spreadsheet

Use the following procedure when printing any spreadsheet.
File
Print
Print Active Sheets (see Fig. 1.13)

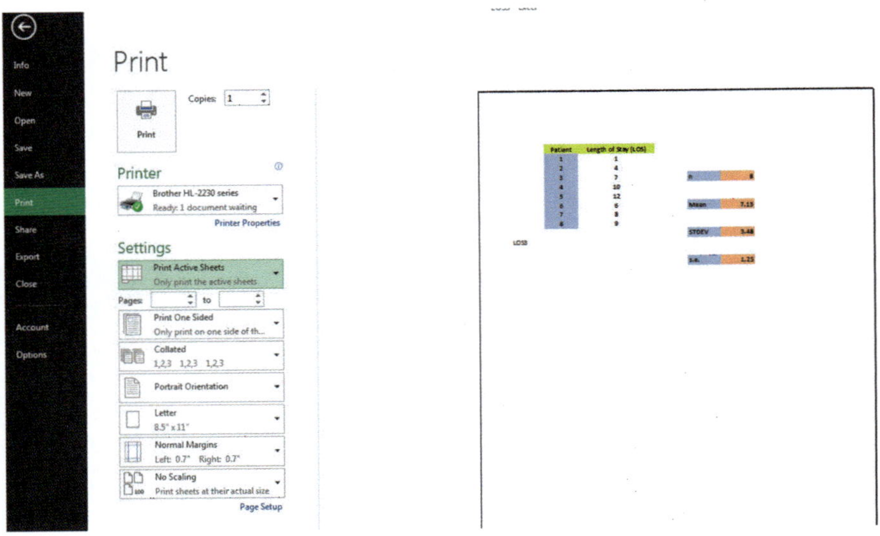

Fig. 1.13 Example of How to Print an Excel Worksheet Using the File/Print/Print Active Sheets Commands

Print (top of your screen)

The final spreadsheet is given in Fig. 1.14

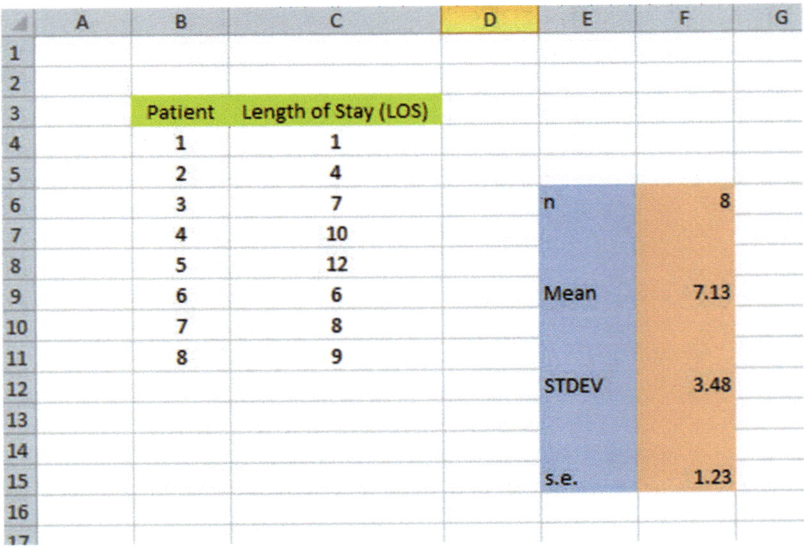

	A	B	C	D	E	F	G
1							
2							
3		Patient	Length of Stay (LOS)				
4		1	1				
5		2	4				
6		3	7		n	8	
7		4	10				
8		5	12				
9		6	6		Mean	7.13	
10		7	8				
11		8	9				
12					STDEV	3.48	
13							
14							
15					s.e.	1.23	
16							
17							

Fig. 1.14 Final Result of Printing an Excel Spreadsheet

Before you leave this chapter, let's practice changing the format of the figures on a spreadsheet with two examples: (1) using two decimal places for figures that are dollar amounts, and (2) using three decimal places for figures.

Save the final spreadsheet by: File/Save, then close your spreadsheet by: File/ Close, and then open a blank Excel spreadsheet by using: File/New/Blank workbook (on the top left of your screen).

1.7 Formatting Numbers in Currency Format (Two Decimal Places)

Objective:	To change the format of figures to dollar format with two decimal places

A3: Price
A4: 1.25
A5: 3.45
A6: 12.95

Highlight cells A4:A6 by left-clicking your mouse on A4 and dragging it down so that these three cells are highlighted in a darker color
Home
Number (top center of screen: click on the down arrow on the right; see Fig. 1.15)

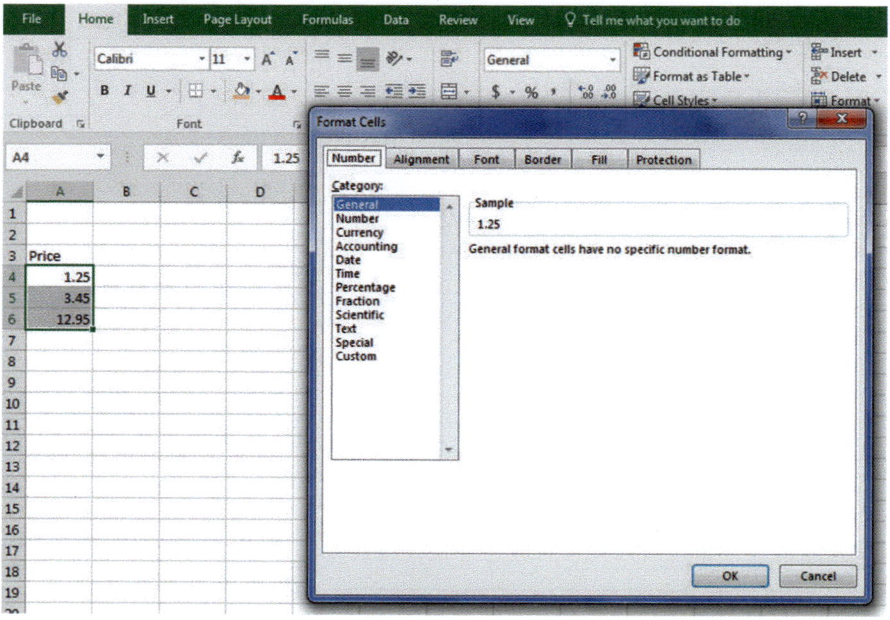

Fig. 1.15 Dialogue Box for Number Format Choices

Category: Currency
Decimal places: 2 (then see Fig. 1.16)

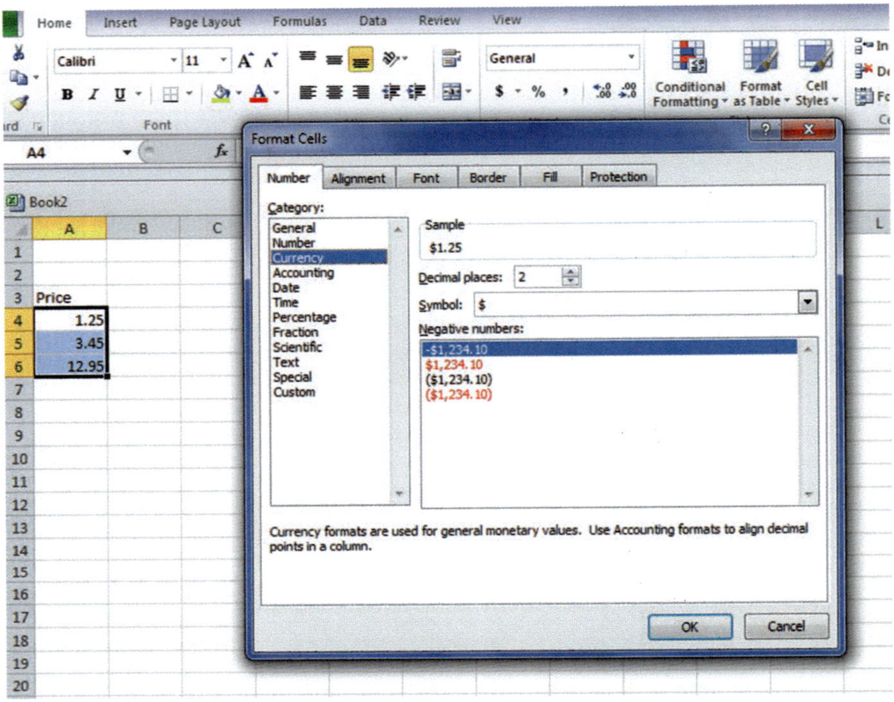

Fig. 1.16 Dialogue Box for Currency (2 decimal places) Format for Numbers

OK

The three cells should have a dollar sign in them and be in two decimal places. Next, let's practice formatting figures in number format, three decimal places.

1.8 Formatting Numbers in Number Format (Three Decimal Places)

Objective: To format figures in number format, three decimal places

Home
Highlight cells A4:A6 on your computer screen
Number (click on the down arrow on the right)
Category: number

At the right of the box, change two decimal places to three decimal places by clicking on the "up arrow" once
OK

The three figures should now be in number format, each with three decimals.

Now, click on any blank cell to deselect cells A4:A6. Then, close this file by File/ Close/Don't Save (since there is no need to save this practice problem).

You can use these same commands to format a range of cells in percentage format (and many other formats) to whatever number of decimal places you want to specify.

1.9 End-of-Chapter Practice Problems

1. An important measurement of the outcome of the residents of homeless shelters is the number of nights spent on the street by each resident in the previous month. Suppose that you recorded this data on 13 residents of a homeless shelter in terms of this statistic. The hypothetical data appear in Fig. 1.17.

Fig. 1.17 Worksheet Data for Chap. 1: Practice Problem #1

RESIDENTS IN A HOMELESS SHELTER

No. of Nights Spent on the Street Last Month

Nights
3
2
1
5
6
4
3
2
7
4
3
5
1

(a) To the right of the table, use Excel to find the sample size, mean, standard deviation, and standard error of the mean for these data. Label your answers, and round off the mean, standard deviation, and standard error of the mean to two decimal places; use number format for these three figures.

(b) Print the result on a separate page.
(c) Save the file as: HOMELESS3

2. Suppose that you have been asked to develop a survey of adoptive parents to determine how the adoption process has been working out for them and for their family. You are in the early stages of developing this survey, but you have decided that Item #12 of the survey will ask the parents to rate the impact of their child's adoption process in their family. You want to try out your Excel skills on a hypothetical set of data for this question. These hypothetical data appear in Fig. 1.18.

ADOPTIVE PARENTS SURVEY						
Item #12:	**"How would you rate the impact of your child's adoption in your family?"**					
1	**2**	**3**	**4**	**5**	**6**	**7**
Very Negative						**Very Positive**
			Data			
			4			
			5			
			3			
			2			
			6			
			7			
			6			
			6			
			5			
			4			
			2			
			5			
			4			
			6			

Fig. 1.18 Worksheet Data for Chap. 1: Practice Problem #2

(a) Use Excel to create a table of these data, and at the right of the table use Excel to find the sample size, mean, standard deviation, and standard error of the mean for these data. Label your answers, and round off the mean, standard deviation, and standard error of the mean to two decimal places using number format.

(b) Print the result on a separate page.
(c) Save the file as: ADOPT3

3. Mental health respite care provides temporary care for individuals with serious mental illnesses who live at home. This type of service provides caregivers with an opportunity to take a break from caregiving without having to worry about the safety of their loved ones. Suppose that you wanted to know the age distribution of patients in such a facility during the past month. The hypothetical data are given in Fig. 1.19:

Fig. 1.19 Worksheet Data for Chap. 1: Practice Problem #3

MENTAL HEALTH RESPITE CARE FACILITY
AGE OF GUESTS
23
26
24
28
31
33
19
25
26
28
29
30
27
24
26

(a) Use Excel to create a table for these data, and at the right of the table, use Excel to find the sample size, mean, standard deviation, and standard error of the mean for these data. Label your answers, and round off the mean, standard deviation, and standard error of the mean to three decimal places using number format.
(b) Print the result on a separate page.
(c) Save the file as: RESPITE3

References

Bowers D. Medical statistics from scratch: an introduction for health professionals. Hoboken: John Wiley & Sons; 2008.

Engel R, Schutt R. The practice of research in social work. 3rd ed. Thousand Oaks CA: SAGE; 2013.

Polit D F. Statistics and data analysis for nursing research. Upper Saddle River: Pearson Education Inc.; 2010.

Schneider R. Basic statistics for social workers. Revised ed. Lanham MD: University Press of America; 2010.

Chapter 2
Random Number Generator

The University of Missouri-St. Louis offers a Bachelor of Social Work (BSW) degree that is fully accredited by the Council on Social Work Education. The program includes a requirement of 570 hours of fieldwork in a social services agency. Suppose that you are the Director of this program and that you want to obtain suggestions as to how the program can be improved from the 32 students who are scheduled to receive their degree in two months. Suppose, further, that you want to take a random sample of 5 of these 32 students so that you can set up a time for a personal interview with each of them.

Using your Excel skills to take this random sample, you will need to define a "sampling frame."

A sampling frame is a list of objects, events, or people from which you want to select a random sample. In this case, it is the group of 32 students in your BSW program. In order to define the sampling frame, you will first assign a unique identifier to each person (or object) in the sampling frame. The frame starts with the identification code (ID) of 1 that is assigned to the first student in the group of 32 students. The second student has a code number of 2, the third a code number of 3, and so forth, until the last student has a code number of 32.

Since the group had 32 students in the BSW program, your sampling frame would go from 1 to 32 with each student having a unique ID number.

We will first create the frame numbers as follows in a new Excel worksheet:

2.1 Creating Frame Numbers for Generating Random Numbers

Objective: To create the frame numbers for generating random numbers

T.J. Quirk, S. Cummings, *Excel 2016 for Social Work Statistics*, Excel for Statistics,
DOI 10.1007/978-3-319-66221-3_2

A3: FRAME NO.
A4: 1

Now, create the frame numbers in column A with the Home/Fill commands that were explained in the first chapter of this book (see Sect. 1.4.1) so that the frame numbers go from 1 to 32, with the number 32 in cell A35. If you need to be reminded about how to do that, here are the steps:

Click on cell A4 to select this cell
Home
Fill (then click on the "down arrow" next to this command and select)
Series (see Fig. 2.1)

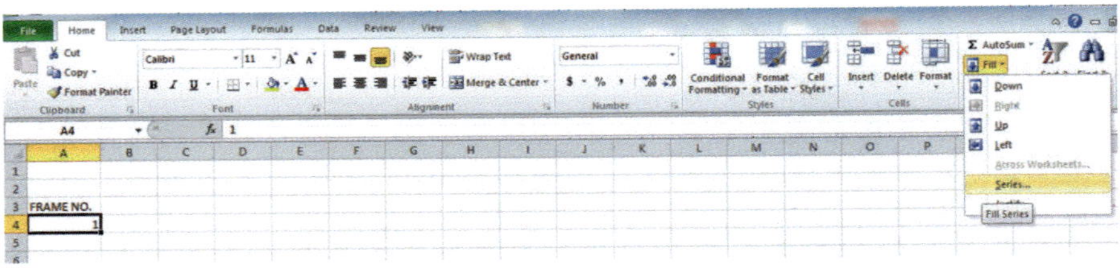

Fig. 2.1 Dialogue Box for Fill/Series Commands

Columns
Step value: 1
Stop value: 32 (see Fig. 2.2)

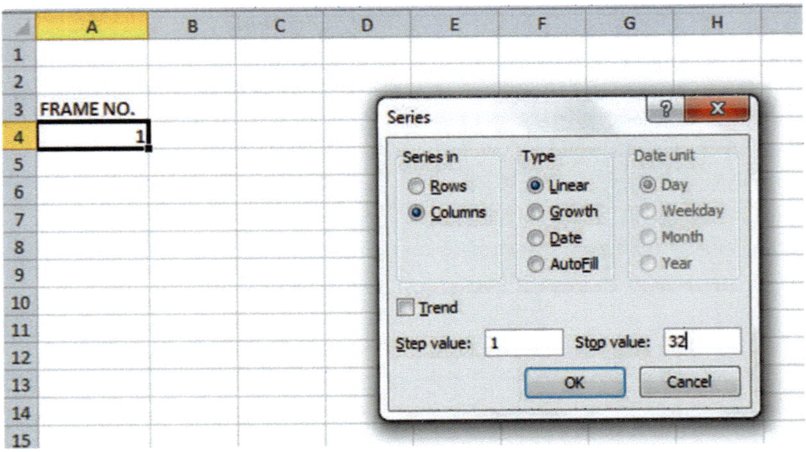

Fig. 2.2 Dialogue Box for Fill/Series/Columns/Step value/Stop value Commands

OK
Then, save this file as: Random29. You should obtain the result in Fig. 2.3.

Fig. 2.3 Frame Numbers from 1 to 32

FRAME NO.
1
2
3
4
5
6
7
8
9
10
11
12
13
14
15
16
17
18
19
20
21
22
23
24
25
26
27
28
29
30
31
32

Now, create a column next to these frame numbers in this manner:

B3: DUPLICATE FRAME NO.
B4: 1

Next, use the Home/Fill command again, so that the 32 frame numbers begin in cell B4 and end in cell B35. Be sure to widen the columns A and B so that all of the information in these columns fits inside the column width. Then, center the information inside both Column A and Column B on your spreadsheet. You should obtain the information given in Fig. 2.4.

Fig. 2.4 Duplicate Frame Numbers from 1 to 32

FRAME NO.	DUPLICATE FRAME NO.
1	1
2	2
3	3
4	4
5	5
6	6
7	7
8	8
9	9
10	10
11	11
12	12
13	13
14	14
15	15
16	16
17	17
18	18
19	19
20	20
21	21
22	22
23	23
24	24
25	25
26	26
27	27
28	28
29	29
30	30
31	31
32	32

Save this file as: Random30

You are probably wondering why you created the same information in both Column A and Column B of your spreadsheet. This is to make sure that before you sort the frame numbers, you have exactly 32 of them when you finish sorting them into a random sequence of 32 numbers.

Now, let's add a random number to each of the duplicate frame numbers as follows:

2.2 Creating Random Numbers in an Excel Worksheet

C3: RANDOM NO.
(then widen columns A, B, C so that their labels fit inside the columns; then center the information in A3:C35)
C4: =RAND()

Next, hit the Enter key to add a random number to cell C4.

Note that you need *both* an open parenthesis *and* a closed parenthesis to create =*RAND*()**.** The RAND command "looks to the left of the cell with the RAND() COMMAND in it" and assigns a random number to that cell.

Now, put the pointer using your mouse in cell C4 and then move the pointer to the bottom right corner of that cell until you see a "plus sign" in that cell. Then, click and drag the pointer down to cell C35 to add a random number to all 32 ID frame numbers (see Fig. 2.5).

Fig. 2.5 Example of Random Numbers Assigned to the Duplicate Frame Numbers

FRAME NO.	DUPLICATE FRAME NO.	RANDOM NO.
1	1	0.178997426
2	2	0.269196787
3	3	0.48649709
4	4	0.882904516
5	5	0.015953504
6	6	0.099651545
7	7	0.42850057
8	8	0.381659988
9	9	0.431296832
10	10	0.476642453
11	11	0.268603728
12	12	0.871330234
13	13	0.775421903
14	14	0.908450998
15	15	0.138749452
16	16	0.159535582
17	17	0.672417279
18	18	0.956231064
19	19	0.486746795
20	20	0.83596565
21	21	0.688574546
22	22	0.467838617
23	23	0.695493167
24	24	0.226521237
25	25	0.335451708
26	26	0.209245145
27	27	0.631291464
28	28	0.210229448
29	29	0.553196562
30	30	0.494647331
31	31	0.986702143
32	32	0.178067956

Then, click on any empty cell to deselect C4:C35 to remove the dark color highlighting these cells.

Save this file as: Random31

Now, let's sort these duplicate frame numbers into a random sequence:

2.3 Sorting Frame Numbers into a Random Sequence

Objective: To sort the duplicate frame numbers into a random sequence

Highlight cells B3: C35 (include the labels at the top of columns B and C)
Data (top of screen)
Sort (click on this word at the top center of your screen; see Fig. 2.6)

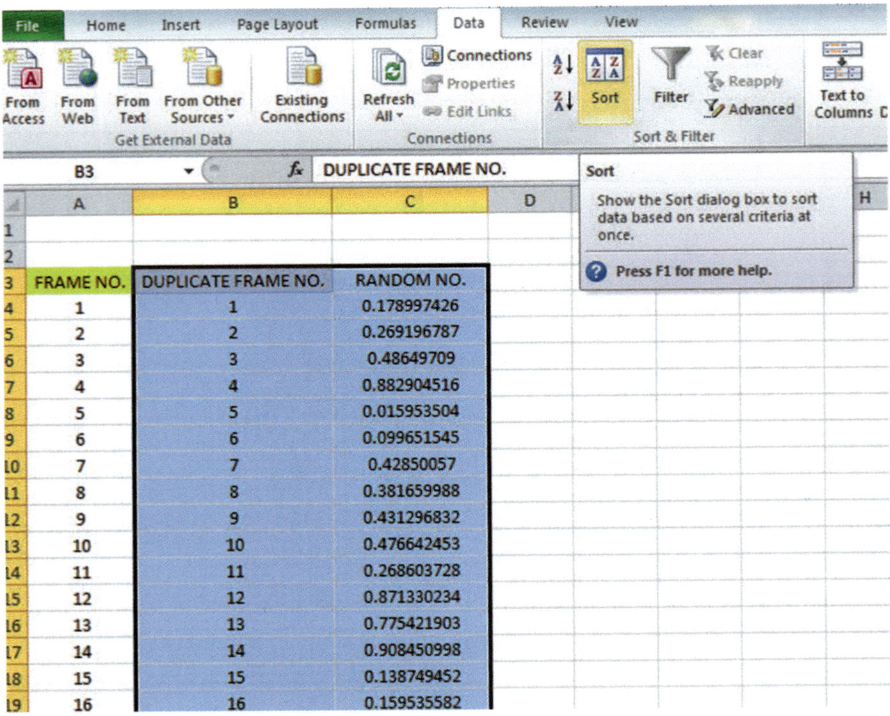

Fig. 2.6 Dialogue Box for Data/Sort Commands

Sort by: RANDOM NO. (click on the down arrow)
Smallest to Largest (see Fig. 2.7)

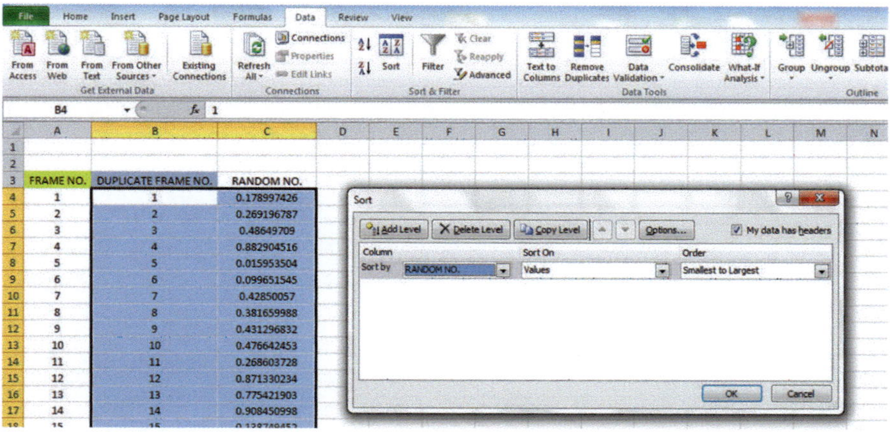

Fig. 2.7 Dialogue Box for Data/Sort/RANDOM NO./Smallest to Largest Commands

OK
Click on any empty cell to deselect B3:C35.
Save this file as: Random32
Print this file now.

These steps will produce Fig. 2.8 with the DUPLICATE FRAME NUMBERS sorted into a random order:

Fig. 2.8 Duplicate Frame Numbers Sorted by Random Number

FRAME NO.	DUPLICATE FRAME NO.	RANDOM NO.
1	5	0.063981403
2	6	0.977468743
3	15	0.225170263
4	16	0.765734052
5	32	0.274680922
6	1	0.594468001
7	26	0.511966171
8	28	0.625577233
9	24	0.906310053
10	11	0.488640116
11	2	0.020129977
12	25	0.723003676
13	8	0.975227547
14	7	0.469582962
15	9	0.14889954
16	22	0.955629903
17	10	0.897398234
18	3	0.314860892
19	19	0.442019486
20	30	0.078566335
21	29	0.172474705
22	27	0.104689528
23	17	0.406630369
24	21	0.961398315
25	23	0.094222677
26	13	0.323429051
27	20	0.470615753
28	12	0.978014724
29	4	0.618082813
30	14	0.727776384
31	18	0.919475329
32	31	0.324497007

Important note: Because Excel randomly assigns these random numbers, your Excel commands will produce a different sequence of random numbers from everyone else who reads this book!

Your objective at the beginning of this chapter was to randomly select 5 of the 32 students in your BSW program. You can now do that by selecting the *first five sorted ID numbers* in the DUPLICATE FRAME NO. column.

Although your first five random numbers will be different from those we have selected in the random sort that we did in this chapter, we would select these five student IDs (see Fig. 2.9).
5, 6, 15, 16, 32

Fig. 2.9 First Five Students Selected Randomly

FRAME NO.	DUPLICATE FRAME NO.	RANDOM NO.
1	5	0.063981403
2	6	0.977468743
3	15	0.225170263
4	16	0.765734052
5	32	0.274680922
6	1	0.594468001
7	26	0.511966171
8	28	0.625577233
9	24	0.906310053
10	11	0.488640116
11	2	0.020129977
12	25	0.723003676
13	8	0.975227547
14	7	0.469582962
15	9	0.14889954
16	22	0.955629903
17	10	0.897398234
18	3	0.314860892
19	19	0.442019486
20	30	0.078566335
21	29	0.172474705
22	27	0.104689528
23	17	0.406630369
24	21	0.961398315
25	23	0.094222677
26	13	0.323429051
27	20	0.470615753
28	12	0.978014724
29	4	0.618082813
30	14	0.727776384
31	18	0.919475329
32	31	0.324497007

Remember, your five ID numbers selected after your random sort will be different from the five ID numbers in Fig. 2.9 because Excel assigns a different random number *each time the =RAND() command is given.*

Before we leave this chapter, you need to learn how to print a file so that all of the information on that file fits onto a single page without "dribbling over" onto a second or third page.

2.4 Printing an Excel File So That All of the Information Fits onto One Page

Objective: To print a file so that all of the information fits onto one page

The three practice problems at the end of this chapter require you to sort random numbers when the files contain 63 social work students, 114 child maltreatment reports, and 75 long-term-care facilities in Missouri, respectively. These files will be "too big" to fit onto one page when you print them unless you format these files so that they fit onto a single page.

Let's create a situation where the file does not fit onto one printed page unless you format it first to do that.

Go back to the file you just created, Random 32, and enter the name: *Jennifer* into cell: A50.

If you printed this file now, the name, *Jennifer*, would be printed onto a second page because it "dribbles over" outside of the page rage for this file in its current format.

So, you would need to change the page format so that all of the information, including the name, Jennifer, fits onto just one page when you print this file by using the following steps:

Click on any empty cell to change the pointer from cell A50
Page Layout (top left of the computer screen)
(Notice the "Scale to Fit" section in the center of your screen; see Fig. 2.10)

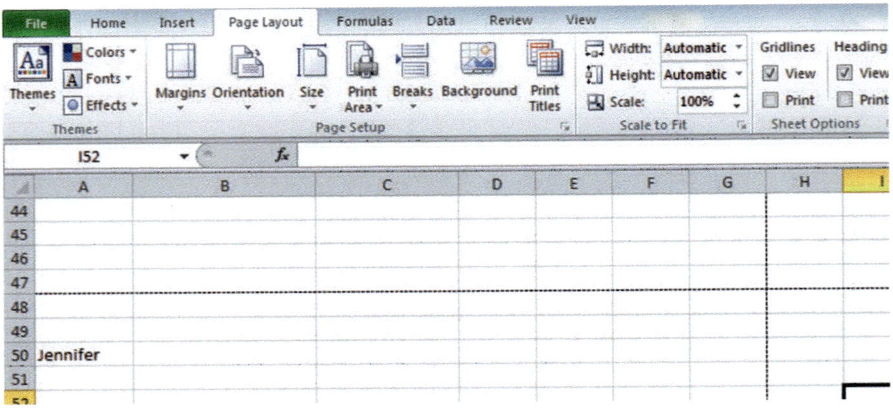

Fig. 2.10 Dialogue Box for Page Layout/Scale to Fit Commands

Hit the down arrow to the right of 100% *once* to reduce the size of the page to 95%

Now, note that the name, Jennifer, is still on a second page on your screen because her name is below the horizontal dotted line on your screen in Fig. 2.11 (the dotted lines tell you outline dimensions of the file if you printed it now).

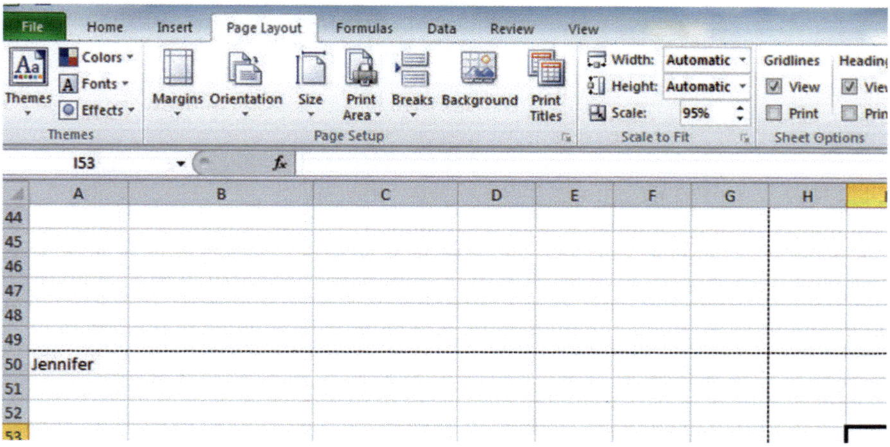

Fig. 2.11 Example of Scale Reduced to 95% with "Jennifer" to be Printed on a Second Page

So, you need to repeat the "scale change steps" by hitting the down arrow on the right once more to reduce the size of the worksheet to 90% of its normal size.

Notice that the "dotted lines" on your computer screen in Fig. 2.12 are now below Jennifer's name to indicate that all of the information, including her name, is now formatted to fit onto just one page when you print this file.

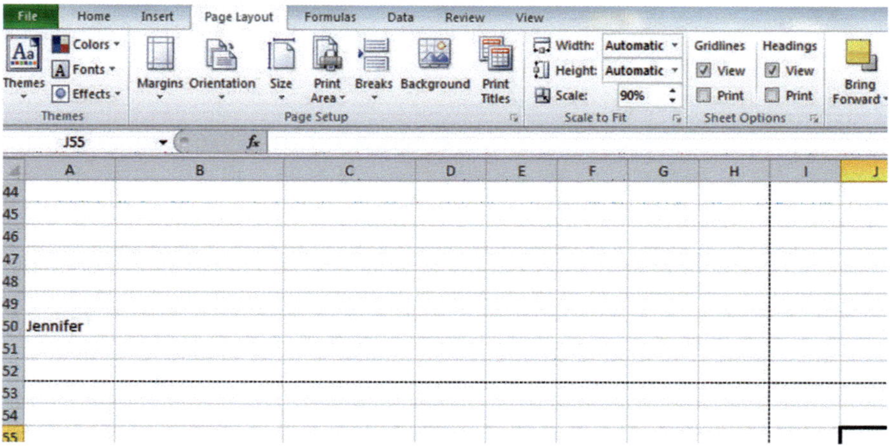

Fig. 2.12 Example of Scale Reduced to 90% with "Jennifer" to be printed on the first page (note the dotted line below Jennifer on your screen)

Save the file as: Random34

Print the file. Does it all fit onto one page? It should (see Fig. 2.13).

Fig. 2.13 Final Spreadsheet of 90% Scale to Fit

FRAME NO.	DUPLICATE FRAME NO.	RANDOM NO.
1	5	0.747176905
2	6	0.038774393
3	15	0.091368861
4	16	0.63147137
5	32	0.190734495
6	1	0.411943765
7	26	0.138033007
8	28	0.927874602
9	24	0.058336576
10	11	0.043243606
11	2	0.729011126
12	25	0.204119693
13	8	0.456656709
14	7	0.232589896
15	9	0.09096704
16	22	0.935399501
17	10	0.201267198
18	3	0.52638312
19	19	0.53734605
20	30	0.969840616
21	29	0.475657455
22	27	0.558049277
23	17	0.488444809
24	21	0.717097206
25	23	0.86192944
26	13	0.875595013
27	20	0.536748908
28	12	0.331784725
29	4	0.642847666
30	14	0.575767804
31	18	0.939789757
32	31	0.776050794
Jennifer		

2.5 End-of-Chapter Practice Problems

1. Suppose that you are the Director of the Master of Social Work (MSW) program at The Brown School at Washington University in St. Louis, MO USA and you want to interview a random sample of students who are scheduled to graduate so that you can obtain their suggestions about how the program can be improved. Assume that 63 students are scheduled to graduate, and that you want to randomly select 15 of these 63 students for a personal interview with you.

   (a) Set up a spreadsheet of frame numbers for these students with the heading: FRAME NUMBERS using the Home/Fill commands.
   (b) Then, create a separate column to the right of these frame numbers which duplicates these frame numbers with the title: Duplicate frame numbers.
   (c) Then, create a separate column to the right of these duplicate frame numbers entitled RANDOM NO. and use the =RAND() function to assign random numbers to all of the frame numbers in the duplicate frame numbers column, and change this column format so that three decimal places appear for each random number.
   (d) Sort the duplicate frame numbers and random numbers into a random order.
   (e) Print the result so that the spreadsheet fits onto one page.
   (f) Circle on your printout the I.D. number of the first 15 students that you would use in your interviews.
   (g) Save the file as: RAND9

   Important note: Note that everyone who does this problem will generate a different random order of ID numbers since Excel assigns a different random number each time the RAND() command is used. For this reason, the answer to the problem given in this Excel Guide will have a completely different sequence of random numbers from the random sequence that you generate. This is normal and what is to be expected.

2. Suppose that a total of 114 child maltreatment reports have been submitted to a state agency in the last month, and that you want to select a random sample of 10 children in this database of reports for case studies.

   (a) Set up a spreadsheet of frame numbers for these claims with the heading: FRAME NO.
   (b) Then, create a separate column to the right of these frame numbers which duplicates these frame numbers with the title: Duplicate frame no.
   (c) Then, create a separate column to the right of these duplicate frame numbers entitled "Random number" and use the =RAND() function to assign random numbers to all of the frame numbers in the duplicate frame numbers column. Then, change this column format so that three decimal places appear for each random number.
   (d) Sort the duplicate frame numbers and random numbers into a random order.

(e) Print the result so that the spreadsheet fits onto one page.
(f) Circle on your printout the I.D. number of the first 10 reports that would be used in this audit.
(g) Save the file as: RANDOM6

3. Suppose, for the sake of argument, that the state of Missouri USA has a total of 75 long-term-care facilities. Assume that you want to randomly sample 20 of the 75 long-term-care facilities to conduct phone interviews with the facility Directors to obtain their ideas as to how you could improve your own organization's care offered to your guests.

(a) Set up a spreadsheet of frame numbers for these facilities with the heading: FRAME NUMBERS.
(b) Then, create a separate column to the right of these frame numbers which duplicates these frame numbers with the title: Duplicate frame numbers
(c) Then, create a separate column to the right of these duplicate frame numbers entitled "Random number" and use the =RAND() function to assign random numbers to all of the frame numbers in the duplicate frame numbers column. Change this column format so that three decimal places appear for each random number.
(d) Sort the duplicate frame numbers and random numbers into a random order.
(e) Print the result so that the spreadsheet fits onto one page.
(f) Circle on your printout the I.D. number of the first 20 facilities that you would select for your phone interviews.
(g) Save the file as: RAND5

Chapter 3
Confidence Interval About the Mean Using the TINV Function and Hypothesis Testing

This chapter focuses on two ideas: (1) finding the 95% confidence interval about the mean, and (2) hypothesis testing.

Let's talk about the confidence interval first and then hypothesis testing.

3.1 Confidence Interval About the Mean

In statistics, we are often interested in *estimating the population mean*. How do we do that?

3.1.1 How to Estimate the Population Mean

Objective: To estimate the population mean, μ

The population mean is an average of all people in a target population. For example, if we were interested in how well adults ages 25–44 liked a new flavor of Ben & Jerry's ice cream, we could never ask this question of all of the people in the U.S. who were in that age group. Such a research study would take way too much time to complete and would be cost prohibitive.

So, instead of testing *everyone* in the population, we take a sample of people in the population and use the results of this sample to estimate the mean of the entire population. This saves both time and money. When we use the results of a sample to estimate the population mean, this is called "*inferential statistics*" because we are inferring the population mean from the sample mean.

T.J. Quirk, S. Cummings, *Excel 2016 for Social Work Statistics*, Excel for Statistics,
DOI 10.1007/978-3-319-66221-3_3

When we study a sample from a population, we know the size of our sample (n), the mean of our sample ($\bar{X}$), and the standard deviation of our sample (STDEV). We use these figures to estimate the accuracy of our estimated population mean with a test called the "confidence interval about the mean."

3.1.2 *Estimating the Lower Limit and the Upper Limit of the 95% Confidence Interval About the Mean*

The theoretical background of this test is beyond the scope of this book, and you can learn more about this test from studying any good statistics textbook (e.g. Veney et al. 2009; Rosenthal 2012) but the basic ideas are as follows.

We assume that the population mean is somewhere in an interval which has a "lower limit" and an "upper limit" to it. We also assume in this book that we want to be "95% confident" that the population mean is inside this interval somewhere. So, we intend to make the following type of statement:

> "We are 95% confident that the population mean of the number of outpatient visits to our clinic during the past 12 months was between 3.25 visits and 3.67 visits."

If we want to claim that the number of outpatient visits to our clinic during the past 12 months was 3.50 visits, we can do this because 3.50 is *inside the 95% confidence interval* in our research study in the above example. We do not know exactly what the population mean is, only that it is somewhere between 3.25 visits and 3.67 visits, and 3.50 visits, which is our sample mean, is inside this interval.

But we are only 95% confident that the population mean is inside this interval, and 5% of the time we will be wrong in assuming that the population mean is 3.50 visits.

For our purposes in science research, we are happy to be 95% confident that our assumption is accurate. We should also point out that 95% is an arbitrary level of confidence for our results. We could choose to be 80% confident, or 90% confident, or even 99% confident in our results if we wanted to do that. In this book, *we will always assume that we want to be 95% confident of our results.* That way, you will not have to guess on how confident you want to be in any of the problems in this book.

So how do we find the 95% confidence interval about the mean for our data?

In words, we will find this interval this way:

> "Take the sample mean ($\bar{X}$), *and add to it* 1.96 times the standard error of the mean (s.e.) to get the upper limit of the confidence interval. Then, take the sample mean, *and subtract from it* 1.96 times the standard error of the mean to get the lower limit of the confidence interval."

You will remember (See Sect. 1.3) that the standard error of the mean (s.e.) is found by dividing the standard deviation of our sample (STDEV) by the square root of our sample size, n.

In mathematical terms, the formula for the 95% confidence interval about the mean is:

$$\bar{X} \pm 1.96 \text{ s.e.} \tag{3.1}$$

Note that the "± *sign*" stands for "plus or minus," and this means that you first add 1.96 times the s.e. of the mean to get the upper limit of the confidence interval, and then subtract 1.96 times the s.e. of the mean to get the lower limit of the confidence interval. Also, the symbol 1.96 s.e. means that you multiply 1.96 times the standard error of the mean to get this part of the formula for the confidence interval.

Note: We will explain shortly where the number 1.96 came from.

Let's try a simple example to illustrate this formula.

3.1.3 Estimating the Confidence Interval for the Number of Outpatient Visits to a Clinic

Let's suppose that you have been asked to conduct a study of outpatient clinic visits. Assume that you took a random sample of 36 patients who required outpatient care in the past 12 months from these clinics and determined that they averaged 3.42 visits to the clinics with a standard deviation of 1.15 visits. The standard error (s.e.) would be 1.15 divided by the square root of 36 (i.e., 6) which gives a s.e. equal to 0.19 visits.

The 95% confidence interval for these data would be:

$$3.42 \pm 1.96\ (0.19)$$

The *upper limit of this confidence interval* uses the plus sign of the ± sign in the formula. Therefore, the upper limit would be:

$$3.42 + 1.96\ (0.19) = 3.42 + 0.37 = 3.79 \text{ visits}$$

Similarly, *the lower limit of this confidence interval* uses the minus sign of the ± sign in the formula. Therefore, the lower limit would be:

$$3.42 - 1.96\ (0.19) = 3.42 - 0.37 = 3.05 \text{ visits}$$

The result of our part of the ongoing research study would, therefore, be the following:

> "We are 95% confident that the population mean for the number of outpatient visits to these clinics during the past 12 months was between 3.05 visits and 3.79 visits."

Based upon the fact that our sample mean of 3.50 visits is inside the confidence interval, we could conclude that the average number of outpatients visits to these clinics in the past 12 months was 3.50 visits. Our data supports this claim because 3.50 visits is inside of this 95% confidence interval for the population mean.

You are probably asking yourself: "Where did that 1.96 in the formula come from?"

3.1.4 Where Did the Number "1.96" Come From?

A detailed mathematical answer to that question is beyond the scope of this book, but here is the basic idea.

We make an assumption that the data in the population are "normally distributed" in the sense that the population data would take the shape of a "normal curve" if we could test all of the people or properties in the population. The normal curve looks like the outline of the Liberty Bell that sits in front of Independence Hall in Philadelphia, Pennsylvania. The normal curve is "symmetric" in the sense that if we cut it down the middle, and folded it over to one side, the half that we folded over would fit perfectly onto the half on the other side.

A discussion of integral calculus is beyond the scope of this book, but essentially we want to find the lower limit and the upper limit of the population data in the normal curve so that 95% of the area under this curve is between these two limits. *If we have more than 40 people in our research study*, the value of these limits is plus or minus 1.96 times the standard error of the mean (s.e.) of our sample. The number 1.96 times the s.e. of our sample gives us the upper limit and the lower limit of our confidence interval. If you want to learn more about this idea, you can consult a good statistics book (e.g. Polit 2010).

The number 1.96 would change if we wanted to be confident of our results at a different level from 95% as long as we have more than 40 people in our research study.

For example:

1. If we wanted to be 80% confident of our results, this number would be 1.282.
2. If we wanted to be 90% confident of our results, this number would be 1.645.
3. If we wanted to be 99% confident of our results, this number would be 2.576.

But since we always want to be 95% confident of our results in this book, we will always use 1.96 in this book whenever we have more than 40 people in our research study.

3.1.5 Finding the Value for t in the Confidence Interval Formula

Objective: To find the value for t in the confidence interval formula

The correct formula for the confidence interval about the mean for different sample sizes is the following:

$$\bar{X} \pm t \text{ s.e.} \qquad (3.2)$$

To use this formula, you find the sample mean, $\bar{X}$, *and add to it the value of t times the s.e. to get the upper limit* of this 95% confidence interval. Also, you take the sample mean $\bar{X}$, and *subtract from it the value of t times the s.e. to get the lower limit* of this 95% confidence interval. And, you find the value of t in the table given in Appendix E of this book in the following way:

Objective: To find the value of t in the t-table in Appendix E

Before we get into an explanation of what is meant by "the value of t," let's give you practice in finding the value of t by using the t-table in Appendix E.

Keep your finger on Appendix E as we explain how you need to "read" that table.

Since the test in this chapter is called the "confidence interval about the mean test," you will use the first column on the left in Appendix E to find the critical value of t for your research study (note that this column is headed: "sample size n").

To find the value of *t* , you go down this first column until you find the sample size in your research study, and then you go to the right and read the value of *t* for that sample size in the "critical t column" of the table (note that this column is the column that you would use for the 95% confidence interval about the mean).

For example, if you have 14 people in your research study, the value of t is 2.160.

If you have 26 people in your research study, the value of t is 2.060.

If you have more than 40 people in your research study, the value of t is always 1.96.

Note that the "critical t column" in Appendix E represents the value of t that you need to use to be 95% confident that your results are "significant".

Throughout this book, we are assuming that you want to be 95% confident in the results of your statistical tests. Therefore, the value for t in the t-table in Appendix E tells you which value you should use for *t* when you use the formula for the 95% confidence interval about the mean.

Now that you know how to find the value of t in the formula for the confidence interval about the mean, let's explore how you find this confidence interval using Excel.

3.1.6 Using Excel's TINV Function to Find the Confidence Interval About the Mean

Objective: To use the TINV function in Excel to find the confidence interval about the mean

When you use Excel, the formulas for finding the confidence interval are:

$$\textit{Lower limit}: \quad = \bar{X} - TINV(1-0.95, n-1)^{*}s.e.(\text{no spaces between these symbols}) \quad (3.3)$$

$$\textit{Upper limit}: \quad = \bar{X} + TINV(1-0.95, n-1)^{*}s.e.(\text{no spaces between these symbols}) \quad (3.4)$$

Note that the "* *symbol*" in this formula tells Excel to use multiplication in the formula, and it stands for "times" in the way we talk about multiplication.

You will recall from Chap. 1 that n stands for the sample size, and so $n - 1$ stands for the sample size minus one.

You will also recall from Chap. 1 that the standard error of the mean, s.e., equals the STDEV divided by the square root of the sample size, n (See Sect. 1.3).

Let's try a sample problem using Excel to find the 95% confidence interval about the mean for a problem.

Let's suppose that a clinic wanted to claim that the average number of outpatient clinic visits during the past 12 months was 3.50 visits. Let's call 3.50 visits the "reference value" for this clinic.

Suppose, further, that you have been asked to check this claim to see if it holds up based on some research evidence. You decide to collect some data and to use the 95% confidence interval about the mean to test your results:

3.1.7 Using Excel to Find the 95% Confidence Interval for a Clinic's Outpatient Visits

Objective: To analyze the data using a 95% confidence interval about the mean

You select a random sample of 25 outpatients and record the number of visits they made to this clinic during these 12 months. Your research study produces the hypothetical results given in Fig. 3.1:

Outpatient Visits
Visits during the past 12 months
2
5
7
4
3
2
4
1
3
2
3
6
5
2
4
3
3
4
6
2
2
3
4
3
2

Fig. 3.1 Worksheet Data for Outpatient Visits (Practical Example)

Create a spreadsheet with these data and use Excel to find the sample size (n), the mean, the standard deviation (STDEV), and the standard error of the mean (s.e.) for these data using the following cell references.

A3: Outpatient Visits
A5: Visits during the past 12 months
A6: 2

Enter the other Outpatient Visits data in cells A7:A30

Now, highlight cells A6:A30 and format these numbers in number format (zero decimal places). Center these numbers in Column A. Then, widen columns A and B by making both of them three times as wide as the original width of column A. Then, widen column C so that it is three times as wide as the original width of column A so that your table looks more professional.

C7: n
C10: Mean
C13: STDEV
C16: s.e.

C19: 95% confidence interval
D21: Lower limit:
D23: Upper limit: (see Fig. 3.2)

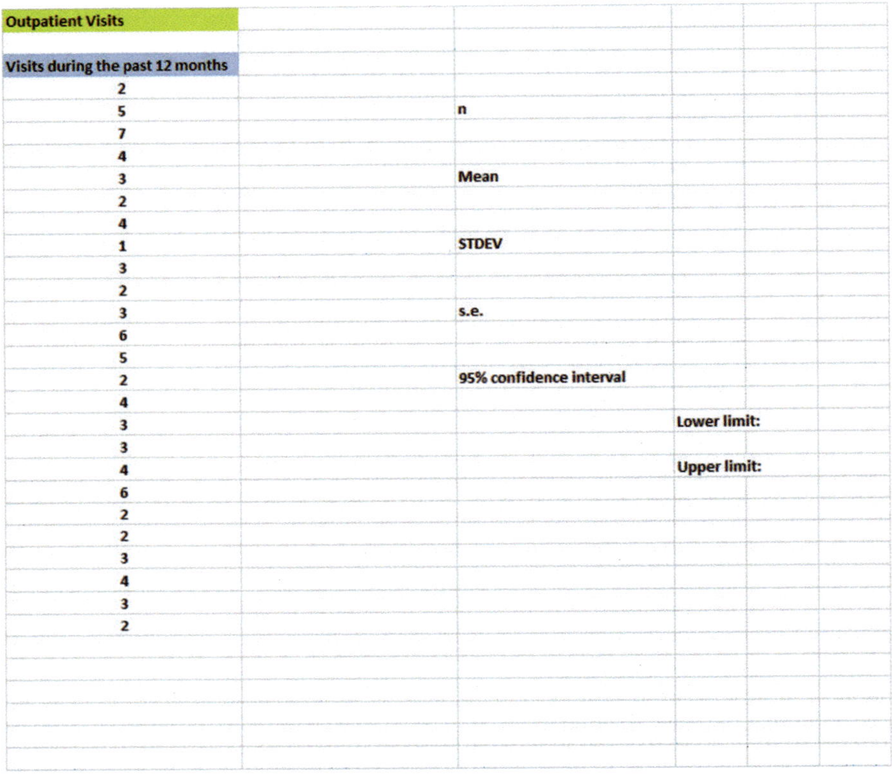

Fig. 3.2 Example of Outpatient Visits Format for the Confidence Interval About the Mean Labels

B26: Draw a picture below this confidence interval
B28: 2.78 (right-align this number)
B29: lower (right-align this word)
B30: limit (right-align this word)
C28: '-------- 3.40 ------- 3.50 ---------- (note that you need to begin cell C28 with a *single quotation mark* (') to tell Excel that this is a *label*, and not a number)
D28: ' ---------- (note the single quotation mark)
E28: 4.02 (left-align this number)
C29: Mean Ref.
C30: value (move to the right under Ref. using the space bar)
E29: upper
E30: limit
B33: Conclusion: (center this word)

Now, align the labels underneath the picture of the confidence interval so that they look like Fig. 3.3.

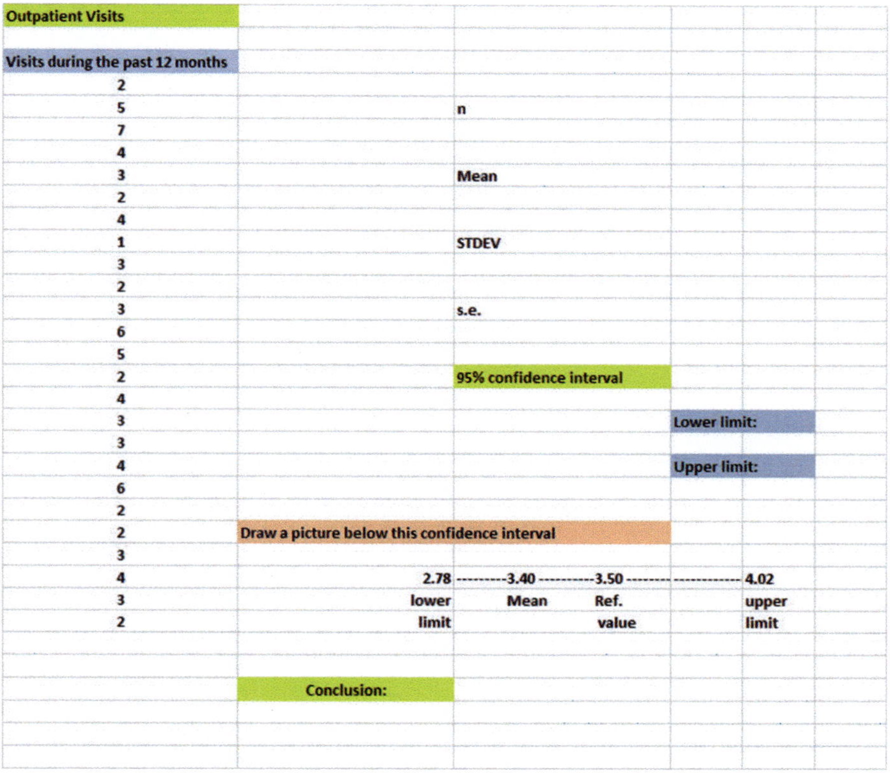

Outpatient Visits					
Visits during the past 12 months					
2					
5		n			
7					
4					
3		Mean			
2					
4					
1		STDEV			
3					
2					
3		s.e.			
6					
5					
2		95% confidence interval			
4					
3			Lower limit:		
3					
4			Upper limit:		
6					
2					
2	Draw a picture below this confidence interval				
3					
4	2.78	---------3.40 ----------3.50 --------	------------	4.02	
3	lower	Mean Ref.		upper	
2	limit	value		limit	
	Conclusion:				

Fig. 3.3 Example of Drawing a Picture of a Confidence Interval About the Mean Result

Next, name the range of data from A6:A30 as: Outpatient4

D7: Use Excel to find the sample size
D10: Use Excel to find the mean
D13: Use Excel to find the STDEV
D16: Use Excel to find the s.e.

Now, you need to find the lower limit and the upper limit of the 95% confidence interval for this study.

We will use Excel's TINV function to do this. We will assume that you want to be 95% confident of your results.

$$\text{F21}: \quad = \text{D10} - \text{TINV}(1 - .95, 24)^{*}\text{D16} \ \ \text{(no spaces between symbols)}$$

Note that this TINV formula uses 24 since 24 is one less than the sample size of 25 (i.e., 24 is n − 1). Note that D10 is the mean, while D16 is the standard error of the mean. The above formula gives the *lower limit of the confidence interval, 2.78.*

$$\text{F23}: \quad = \text{D10} + \text{TINV}(1 - .95, 24)^{*}\text{D16} \ \text{(no spaces between symbols)}$$

The above formula gives the *upper limit of the confidence interval, 4.02.*

Now, use number format (two decimal places) in your Excel spreadsheet for the mean, standard deviation, standard error of the mean, and for both the lower limit and the upper limit of your confidence interval. If you printed this spreadsheet now, the lower limit of the confidence interval (2.78) and the upper limit of the confidence interval (4.02) would “dribble over” onto a second printed page because the information on the spreadsheet is too large to fit onto one page in its present format.

So, you need to use Excel’s “Scale to Fit” commands that we discussed in Chap. 2 (see Sect. 2.4) to reduce the size of the spreadsheet to 80% of its current size using the Page Layout/Scale to Fit function. Do that now, and notice that the dotted line to the right of 2.78 and 4.02 indicates that these numbers would now fit onto one page when the spreadsheet is printed out (see Fig. 3.4)

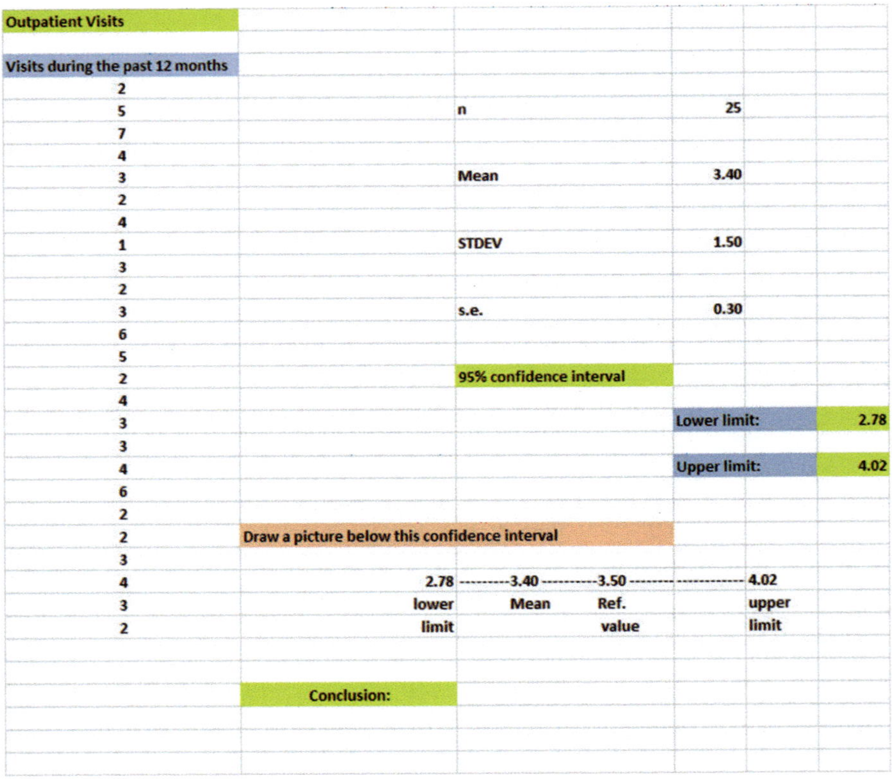

Fig. 3.4 Result of Using the TINV Function to Find the Confidence Interval About the Mean

Note that you have drawn a picture of the 95% confidence interval beneath cell B26, including the lower limit, the upper limit, the mean, and the reference value of 3.50.

Now, let's write the conclusion to your research study on your spreadsheet:

C33: Since the reference value of 3.50 is inside the
C34: confidence interval, we accept that the average
C35: number of outpatient visits to the clinic during
C36: the past 12 months was 3.50 visits.

Important note: You are probably wondering why we wrote the conclusion on four separate lines of the spreadsheet instead of writing it on one long line. This is because if you wrote it on one line, two things would happen that you would not like: (1) If you printed the conclusion by reducing the size of the layout of the page so that the entire spreadsheet would fit onto one page, the print font size for the entire spreadsheet would be so small that you could not read it without a magnifying glass, and (2) If you printed the spreadsheet without reducing the page size layout, it would "dribble over" part of the conclusion to a separate page all by itself, and your spreadsheet would not look professional.

Your research study accepted the claim that the average number of outpatients visits to the clinic during the past 12 months was 3.50 visits. (See Fig. 3.5)

Outpatient Visits					
Visits during the past 12 months					
2					
5		**n**	**25**		
7					
4					
3		**Mean**	**3.40**		
2					
4					
1		**STDEV**	**1.50**		
3					
2					
3		**s.e.**	**0.30**		
6					
5					
2		**95% confidence interval**			
4					
3			**Lower limit:**		**2.78**
3					
4			**Upper limit:**		**4.02**
6					
2					
2	**Draw a picture below this confidence interval**				
3					
4	**2.78**	**------------3.40-----3.50---------**	**--------------**	**4.02**	
3	**lower**	**Mean Ref.**		**upper**	
2	**limit**	**value**		**limit**	
	Conclusion:	**Since the reference value of 3.50 is inside the**			
		confidence interval, we accept that the average			
		number of outpatient visits to the clinic during			
		the past 12 months was 3.50 visits.			

Fig. 3.5 Final Spreadsheet for the Outpatient Visits Confidence Interval About the Mean

Save your resulting spreadsheet as: **OUTPATIENT3**

3.2 Hypothesis Testing

One of the important activities of research scientists is that they attempt to "check" their assumptions about the world by testing these assumptions in the form of hypotheses.

A typical hypothesis is in the form: *"If x , then y."*

Some examples would be:

1. "If we use this new method of conducting this type of procedure in the laboratory, the cost of completing this procedure will decrease by 3 percent."
2. "If we change the way we teach the online Health Care Law course in our program, then we will obtain a five percent increase in course enrollment."
3. "If we change the format for teaching Advanced Research Methods to graduate students in our MSW program, then their final exam scores will increase by 8 percent."

A hypothesis, then, to a research scientist is a "guess" about what we think is true in the real world. We can test these guesses using statistical formulas to see if our predictions come true.

So, in order to perform these statistical tests, we must first state our hypotheses so that we can test our results against our hypotheses to see if our hypotheses match reality.

So, how do we generate hypotheses in our research?

3.2.1 Hypotheses Always Refer to the Population That You Are Studying

The first step is to understand that our hypotheses always refer to the *population* of people or events in a study.

For example, suppose we are interested in evaluating our social work MSW program by using an in-depth interview with students two months before they are scheduled to graduate from the program. If we select a random sample of students to be interviewed, the selected students would be our sample. This sample would then be used to generalize our findings to the population of all students scheduled to graduate in two months from this program.

All of the students scheduled to graduate from this program in two months would be the *population* that we are interested in studying, while the specific students interviewed in our study would be called the *sample* from this population.

Since our sample sizes typically contain only a portion of the population we are interested in studying, we are interested in the results of our sample *only insofar as the results of our sample can be "generalized" to the population in which we are really interested.*

That is why our hypotheses always refer to the population, and never to the sample of people or events in our study.

You will recall from Chap. 1 that we used the symbol: $\bar{X}$ to refer to the mean of the sample we use in our research study (See Sect. 1.1).

We will use the symbol: μ (the Greek letter "mu") to refer to the *population mean.*

In testing our hypotheses, we are trying to decide which one of two competing hypotheses *about the population mean* we should accept given our data set.

3.2.2 The Null Hypothesis and the Research (Alternative) Hypothesis

These two competing hypotheses are called the *null hypothesis* and the *research hypothesis.*

Statistics textbooks typically refer to the *null hypothesis* with the notation: $H_{0.}$

The *research hypothesis* is typically referred to with the notation: H_1, and it is sometimes called the *alternative hypothesis.*

Let's explain first what is meant by the null hypothesis and the research hypothesis:

(1) *The null hypothesis is what we accept as true unless we have compelling evidence that it is not true.*
(2) *The research hypothesis is what we accept as true whenever we reject the null hypothesis as true.*

This is similar to our legal system in America where we assume that a supposed criminal is innocent until he or she is proven guilty in the eyes of a jury. Our null hypothesis is that this defendant is innocent, while the research hypothesis is that he or she is guilty.

In the great state of Missouri, every license plate has the state slogan: "Show me." This means that people in Missouri think of themselves as not gullible enough to accept everything that someone says as true unless that person's actions indicate the truth of his or her claim. In other words, people in Missouri believe strongly that a person's actions speak much louder than that person's words.

Since both the null hypothesis and the research hypothesis cannot both be true, the task of hypothesis testing using statistical formulas is to decide which one you will accept as true.

Sometimes in social work research studies, rating scales are used in surveys to measure people's attitudes toward an organization's activities. These rating scales are typically 5-point, 7-point, or 10-point scales, although other scale values may also be used.

3.2.2.1 Determining the Null Hypothesis and the Research Hypothesis When Rating Scales Are Used

The following examples are a way to test the null hypothesis and research hypothesis using rating scales. They illustrate how you would test these hypotheses if you encountered rating scales on your job.

The American Health Information Management Association (AHIMA) has more than 67,000 members who work in a variety of health information settings that connect clinical, operational, and administrative functions.

Here is a typical example of a 7-point scale that could be used by the American Health Information Management Association (AHIMA) to obtain feedback from participants on the value of its annual week-long international conference (see Fig. 3.6):

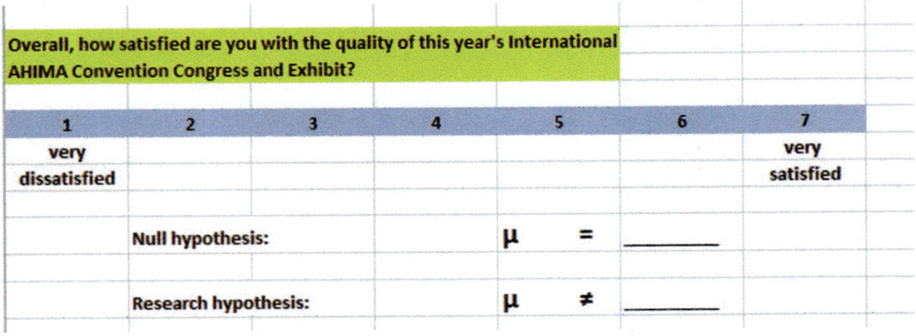

Fig. 3.6 Example of a Rating Scale Item for a Conference (Practical Example)

So, how do we decide what to use as the null hypothesis and the research hypothesis whenever rating scales are used?

Objective: To decide on the null hypothesis and the research hypothesis whenever rating scales are used.

In order to make this determination, we will use a simple rule:

Rule: Whenever rating scales are used, we will use the "middle" of the scale as the null hypothesis and the research hypothesis.

In the above example, since 4 is the number in the middle of the scale (i.e., three numbers are below it, and three numbers are above it), our hypotheses become:

Null hypothesis: $\mu = 4$
Research hypothesis: $\mu \neq 4$

In the above rating scale example, if the result of our statistical test for this one attitude scale item indicates that our population mean is "close to 4," we say that we accept the null hypothesis that the AHIMA conference participants were neither satisfied nor dissatisfied with the overall quality of the conference.

In the above example, *if the result of our statistical test indicates that the population mean is significantly different from 4*, we reject the null hypothesis and accept the research hypothesis *by stating either that*:

"*AHIMA conference participants were significantly satisfied with the overall quality of the conference*" (this is true whenever our sample mean is significantly greater than our expected population mean of 4).

or

"*AHIMA conference participants were significantly dissatisfied with the overall quality of the conference*" (this is accepted as true whenever our sample mean is significantly less than our expected population mean of 4).

Both of these conclusions cannot be true. We accept one of the hypotheses as "true" based on the data set in our research study, and the other one as "not true" based on our data set.

The job of the researcher, then, is to decide which of these two hypotheses, the null hypothesis or the research hypothesis, he or she will accept as true given the data set in the research study.

Let's try some examples of rating scales so that you can practice figuring out what the null hypothesis and the research hypothesis are for each rating scale.

In the spaces in Fig. 3.7, write in the null hypothesis and the research hypothesis for the rating scales:

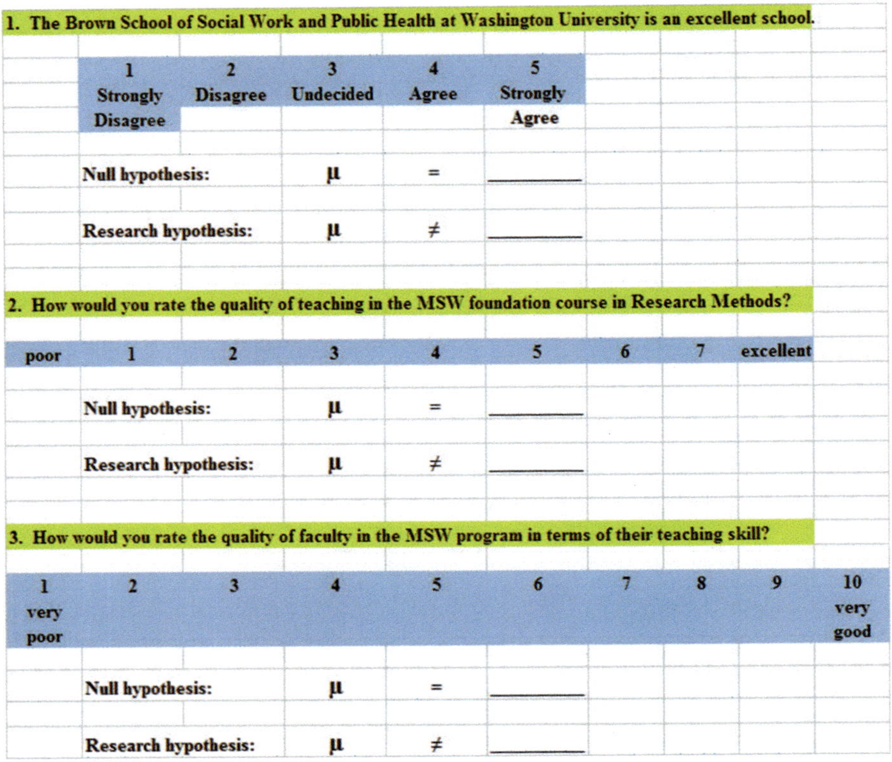

Fig. 3.7 Examples of Rating Scales for Determining the Null Hypothesis and the Research Hypothesis

How did you do?

Here are the answers to these three questions:

1. The null hypothesis is $\mu = 3$, and the research hypothesis is $\mu \neq 3$ on this 5-point scale (i.e. the "middle" of the scale is 3).
2. The null hypothesis is $\mu = 4$, and the research hypothesis is $\mu \neq 4$ on this 7-point scale (i.e., the "middle" of the scale is 4).
3. The null hypothesis is $\mu = 5.5$, and the research hypothesis is $\mu \neq 5.5$ on this 10-point scale (i.e., the "middle" of the scale is 5.5 since there are 5 numbers below 5.5 and 5 numbers above 5.5).

As another example, Webster University, whose main campus is in St. Louis, Missouri USA, uses a Course Feedback form for student evaluations at the end of all of its courses which are offered to more than 16,000 students in 60 cities and 11 countries. The Course Feedback form has 12 rating items referring to the course's planning and organization and the level of communications between the instructor and the students. The ratings are summarized and the results given to instructors after the course is completed. Each of the items is rated on the following 4-point scale:

1 = Very Effective
2 = Effective
3 = Ineffective
4 = Very Ineffective

On this scale, the null hypothesis is: $\mu = 2.5$ and the research hypothesis is: $\mu \neq 2.5$, because there are two numbers below 2.5, and two numbers above 2.5 on the rating scale. (Note that the scale is scored so that a low score, like a low score in golf, is a better score.)

Now, let's discuss the 7 STEPS of hypothesis testing for using the confidence interval about the mean.

3.2.3 The 7 Steps for Hypothesis-Testing Using the Confidence Interval About the Mean

Objective: To learn the 7 steps of hypothesis-testing using the confidence interval about the mean

There are seven basic steps of hypothesis-testing for this statistical test.

3.2.3.1 STEP 1: State the Null Hypothesis and the Research Hypothesis

If you are using numerical scales in your survey, you need to remember that the null and research hypotheses refer to the "middle" of the numerical scale. For example, if you are using 7-point scales with 1 = poor and 7 = excellent, these hypotheses would refer to the middle of these scales and would be:

Null hypothesis H_0: $\mu = 4$
Research hypothesis H_1: $\mu \neq 4$

3.2.3.2 STEP 2: Select the Appropriate Statistical Test

In this chapter we are studying the confidence interval about the mean, and so we will select that test.

3.2.3.3 STEP 3: Calculate the Formula for the Statistical Test

You will recall (see Sect. 3.1.5) that the formula for calculating the confidence interval about the mean is:

$$\bar{X} \pm \text{t s.e.} \tag{3.2}$$

We discussed the procedure for computing this formula for the confidence interval about the mean using Excel earlier in this chapter. The steps involved in using that formula are:

1. Use Excel's =COUNT function to find the sample size.
2. Use Excel's =AVERAGE function to find the sample mean, $\bar{X}$.
3. Use Excel's =STDEV function to find the standard deviation, STDEV.
4. Find the standard error of the mean (s.e.) by dividing the standard deviation (STDEV) by the square root of the sample size, n.
5. Use Excel's TINV function to find the lower limit of the confidence interval.
6. Use Excel's TINV function to find the upper limit of the confidence interval.

3.2.3.4 STEP 4: Draw a Picture of the Confidence Interval About the Mean, Including the Mean, the Lower Limit of the Interval, the Upper Limit of the Interval, and the Reference Value Given in the Null Hypothesis, H_0 (We Will Explain Step 4 Later in the Chapter)

3.2.3.5 STEP 5: Decide on a Decision Rule

(a) *If the reference value is inside the confidence interval, accept the null hypothesis, H_0*
(b) *If the reference value is outside the confidence interval, reject the null hypothesis, H_0, and accept the research hypothesis, H_1*

3.2.3.6 STEP 6: State the Result of Your Statistical Test

There are two possible results when you use the confidence interval about the mean, and only one of them can be accepted as "true." So your result would be one of the following:

Either: Since the reference value is inside the confidence interval, *we accept the null hypothesis, H_0*

Or: Since the reference value is outside the confidence interval, *we reject the null hypothesis, H_0, and accept the research hypothesis, H_1*

3.2.3.7 STEP 7: State the Conclusion of Your Statistical Test in Plain English!

In practice, this is more difficult than it sounds because you are trying to summarize the result of your statistical test in simple English that is both concise and accurate so that someone who has never had a statistics course (such as your boss, perhaps) can understand the conclusion of your test. This is a difficult task, and we will give you lots of practice doing this last and most important step throughout this book.

Objective: To write the conclusion of the confidence interval about the mean test

Let's set some basic rules for stating the conclusion of a hypothesis test.

Rule #1: Whenever you reject H_0 and accept H_1, you must use the word "significantly" in the conclusion to alert the reader that this test found an important result.

Rule #2: Create an outline in words of the "key terms" you want to include in your conclusion so that you do not forget to include some of them.

Rule #3: Write the conclusion in plain English so that the reader can understand it even if that reader has never taken a statistics course.

Let's practice these rules using the outpatient visits Excel spreadsheet that you created earlier in this chapter (OUTPATIENT3), .but first we need to state the hypotheses for that clinic.

If the clinic wants to claim that the average number of outpatient visits during the past 12 months was 3.50 visits, the hypotheses would be:

H_0 : $\mu = 3.50$ visits
H_1 : $\mu \neq 3.50$ visits

You will remember that the reference value of 3.50 was inside the 95% confidence interval about the mean for your data, so we would accept H_0 that the average number of outpatient visits to the clinic during the past 12 months was 3.50.

Objective: To state the result when you accept H_0

Result: Since the reference value of 3.50 is inside the confidence interval, we accept the null hypothesis, H_0.

Let's try our three rules now:

Objective: To write the conclusion when you accept H_0

Rule #1: *Since the reference value was inside the confidence interval, we cannot use the word "significantly" in the conclusion. This is a basic rule we are using in this chapter for every problem.*

Rule #2: The key terms in the conclusion would be:

– outpatient visits
– clinic
– during the past 12 months
– average number
– 3.50 visits

Rule #3: The average number of outpatient visits to the clinic during the past 12 months was 3.50 visits.

The process of writing the conclusion when you accept H_0 is relatively straightforward since you put into words what you said when you wrote the null hypothesis.

However, the process of stating the conclusion when you reject H_0 and accept H_1 is more difficult, so let's practice writing that type of conclusion with three practice case examples:

Objective: To write the result and conclusion when you reject H_0

CASE #1: Suppose that your organization did a time and motion study several months ago of a specific laboratory procedure and determined that the average time required (to the nearest minute) to complete this procedure was 25 minutes. The hypotheses would be:

$H_0: \quad \mu = 25$ minutes
$H_1: \quad \mu \neq 25$ minutes

Suppose that your research yields the following confidence interval:

19	21	23	25
lower limit	Mean	upper limit	Ref. Value

Result: Since the reference value is outside the confidence interval, we reject the null hypothesis and accept the research hypothesis

The three rules for stating the conclusion would be:

Rule #1: We must include the word "significantly" since the reference value of 25 is outside the confidence interval.

Rule #2: The key terms would be:

– laboratory procedure
– average time needed to complete the procedure

– significantly
– either "more than" or "less than"
– and probably closer to

Rule #3: The average laboratory time needed to complete this procedure was significantly less than 25 minutes, and it was probably closer to 21 minutes (i.e., the sample mean).

Note that this conclusion says that the time needed to complete the procedure was less than 25 minutes because the sample mean was only 21 minutes. Note, also, that when you find a significant result by rejecting the null hypothesis, *it is not sufficient to say only: "significantly less than 25 minutes,"* because that does not tell the reader "how much less than 25 minutes" the sample mean was from 25 minutes. To make the conclusion clear, you need to add: "probably closer to 21 minutes" since the sample mean was only 21 minutes.

CASE #2: A health care center typically has hundreds, if not thousands, of patient discharges during a given year. If a financial officer wants to find out the cost of the services provided to a patient, he or she could select a random sample of the discharges during the past year and use it to estimate the true cost of patient care. Let's suppose that the center has determined that the typical cost of patients treated for the same type of disorder and who were discharged during the past year has been $5,642.

You want to practice your data interpretation skills on the hypothetical data which produces the confidence interval below:

The hypotheses for this test would be:

$$H_0: \quad \mu = \$5,642$$
$$H_1: \quad \mu \neq \$5,642$$

Essentially, the null hypothesis states that if the obtained average cost for this sample is not significantly different from $5,642, then it is reasonable to assume that the true cost of this procedure is $5,642.

Suppose that your analysis produced the following confidence interval for this test:

$5,555	$5,584	$5,613	$5,642
lower limit	Mean	upper limit	Ref. Value

Result: Since the reference value is outside the confidence interval, we reject the null hypothesis and accept the research hypothesis.

Rule #1: You must include the word "significantly" since the reference value is outside the confidence interval

Rule #2: The key terms would be:

- average cost
- patients discharged
- during the past year
- for a specific disorder
- significantly
- less or greater (depending on your result)

Rule #3: The average cost of patients discharged during the past year who were treated for a specific disorder was significantly less than \$5,642, and was probably closer to \$5,584.

Note that you need to use the word "less" since the sample mean of \$5,584 was less than the reference value of \$5,642.

CASE #3: The American College of Healthcare Executives (ACHE) has more than 40,000 healthcare professionals in its international membership. ACHE is known for its magazine (*Healthcare Executive*) and for its career development and public policy activities. ACHE sends a survey to a sample of its members, and one of the key questions on the survey asks members whether they agree or disagree that the professional relationships they have formed through ACHE have been important to their career. Members are asked to rate their opinion on a scale where Strongly Disagree is scored as 1, Disagree is scored as 2, Neutral is scored as 3, Agree is scored as 4, and Strongly Agree is scored as 5.

Suppose that you have been asked to use your Excel skills to determine the opinion of the sampled members.

The hypotheses would be:

$H_0: \quad \mu = 3$

$H_1: \quad \mu \neq 3$

Suppose that your research produced the following confidence interval for this survey item:

3	3.4	3.6	3.8
Ref. Value	lower limit	Mean	upper limit

Result: Since the reference value is outside the confidence interval, we reject the null hypothesis and accept the research hypothesis

The three rules for stating the conclusion would be:

Rule #1: You must include the word "significantly" since the reference value is outside the confidence interval

Rule #2: The key terms would be:

- members of ACHE sampled
- professional relationships
- through ACHE membership
- important to their careers
- significantly
- agreed or disagreed

Rule #3: The sample of members of ACHE significantly agreed that the professional relationships they developed through ACHE membership have been important to their careers.

Important note: In this case, you should not use the phrase: "and was probably closer to 3.6" because words can be accurately used to summarize the conclusion without needing to refer to any numbers.

If you want a more detailed explanation of the confidence interval about the mean, see Veney (2003) and Weinbach (2010).

The three practice problems at the end of this chapter will give you additional practice in stating the conclusion of your result, and this book will include many more examples that will help you to write a clear and accurate conclusion to your research findings.

3.3 Alternative Ways to Summarize the Result of a Hypothesis Test

It is important for you to understand that in this book we are summarizing an hypothesis test in one of two ways: (1) We accept the null hypothesis, or (2) We reject the null hypothesis and accept the research hypothesis. We are consistent in the use of these words so that you can understand the concept underlying hypothesis testing.

However, there are many other ways to summarize the result of an hypothesis test, and all of them are correct theoretically, even though the terminology differs. If you are taking a course with a professor who wants you to summarize the results of a statistical test of hypotheses in language which is different from the language we are using in this book, do not panic! If you understand the concept of hypothesis testing as described in this book, you can then translate your understanding to use the terms that your professor wants you to use to reach the same conclusion.

Statisticians and statistics professors of social work all have their own language that they like to use to summarize the results of a hypothesis test. There is no one set of words that these statisticians and professors will ever agree on, and so we have chosen the one that we believe to be easier to understand in terms of the concept of hypothesis testing.

To convince you that there are many ways to summarize the results of a hypothesis test, we present the following quotes from prominent statistics and research books to give you an idea of the different ways that are possible.

3.3.1 *Different Ways to Accept the Null Hypothesis*

The following quotes are typical of the language used in statistics and research books *when the null hypothesis is accepted*:

"The null hypothesis is not rejected." (Black 2010, p. 310)
"The null hypothesis cannot be rejected." (McDaniel and Gates 2010, p. 545)
"The null hypothesis . . . claims that there is no difference between groups." (Salkind 2010, p. 193)
"The difference is not statistically significant." (McDaniel and Gates 2010, p. 545)
" . . . the obtained value is not extreme enough for us to say that the difference between Groups 1 and 2 occurred by anything other than chance." (Salkind 2010, p. 225)
"If we do not reject the null hypothesis, we conclude that there is not enough statistical evidence to infer that the alternative (hypothesis) is true." (Keller 2009, p. 358)
"The research hypothesis is not supported." (Zikmund and Babin 2010, p. 552)

3.3.2 *Different Ways to Reject the Null Hypothesis*

The following quotes are typical of the quotes used in statistics and research books *when the null hypothesis is rejected*:

"The null hypothesis is rejected." (McDaniel and Gates 2010, p. 546)
"If we reject the null hypothesis, we conclude that there is enough statistical evidence to infer that the alternative hypothesis is true." (Keller 2009, p. 358)
"If the test statistic's value is inconsistent with the null hypothesis, we reject the null hypothesis and infer that the alternative hypothesis is true." (Keller 2009, p. 348)
"Because the observed value . . . is greater than the critical value . . ., the decision is to reject the null hypothesis." (Black 2010, p. 359)
"If the obtained value is more extreme than the critical value, the null hypothesis cannot be accepted." (Salkind 2010, p. 243)
"The critical t-value . . . must be surpassed by the observed t-value if the hypothesis test is to be statistically significant . . .." (Zikmund and Babin 2010, p. 567)
"The calculated test statistic . . . exceeds the upper boundary and falls into this rejection region. The null hypothesis is rejected." (Weiers 2011, p. 330)

You should note that all of the above quotes are used by statisticians and professors when discussing the results of a hypothesis test, and so you should not be surprised if someone asks you to summarize the results of a statistical test using different language than we are using in this book.

3.4 End-of-Chapter Practice Problems

1. Royse (2010) discusses an outcome instrument for assessing the results of a social service program. The Rosenberg Self-Esteem Scale was originally developed on high school juniors and seniors. This scale is in the public domain and

may be used without the need for permission. The scale consists of ten items that are each scored on the following 4-point scale:

4 = Strongly Agree
3 = Agree
2 = Disagree
1 = Strongly Disagree

If the ten items are summed, the total score can range from 10 to 40 such that the higher the summed score, the higher the self-esteem. Suppose that you wanted to test your Excel skills on just one item of this scale: "Item 10: I take a positive attitude toward myself." You have decided to create some data from a recently completed drug treatment program for high school seniors to determine their measure of self-esteem. Some hypothetical data are presented in Fig. 3.8.

SELF-ESTEEM MEASURE OF HIGH SCHOOL SENIORS			
DRUG TREATMENT PROGRAM OUTCOME MEASURE			
Item #10:	**"I take a positive attitude toward myself."**		
4	**3**	**2**	**1**
Strongly Agree	**Agree**	**Disagree**	**Strongly Disagree**
	RATING		
	4		
	2		
	3		
	2		
	4		
	3		
	3		
	4		
	4		
	1		
	3		
	4		
	4		
	3		
	4		

Fig. 3.8 Worksheet Data for Chap. 3: Practice Problem #1

(a) To the right of this table, use Excel to find the sample size, mean, standard deviation, and standard error of the mean for the self-esteem figures. Label your answers. Use number format (one decimal place) for the mean, standard deviation, and standard error of the mean.
(b) Enter the null hypothesis and the research hypothesis onto your spreadsheet.
(c) Use Excel's TINV function to find the 95% confidence interval about the mean for these figures. Label your answers. Use number format (one decimal place).
(d) Enter your *result* onto your spreadsheet.
(e) Enter your *conclusion in plain English* onto your spreadsheet.
(f) Print the final spreadsheet to fit onto one page (if you need help remembering how to do this, see the objectives at the end of Chap. 2 in Sect. 2.4)
(g) On your printout, draw a diagram of this 95% confidence interval by hand
(h) Save the file as: selfesteem3

2. Suppose that a residential elder care organization in Missouri wants to obtain feedback about the quality of its website that describes the services offered by this organization in various parts of the state. You are in the early stages of developing an online survey of ten items that can be administered to visitors to the organization's website, but you want to be sure that a key question is asked about the satisfaction of visitors with the website. Let's suppose that you have taken a small random sample of visitors and that you want to analyze the hypothetical data from Item #10 in Fig. 3.9.

RESIDENTIAL ELDER CARE CHAIN IN MISSOURI									
Item #10: How satisfied are you with the Elder Care current website?									
1	2	3	4	5	6	7	8	9	10
Not at all satisfied									Very satisfied
	RATING								
	4								
	6								
	5								
	7								
	8								
	3								
	4								
	5								
	3								
	2								
	4								
	3								
	5								
	7								
	6								
	4								
	3								
	7								
	8								
	5								
	6								
	4								
	3								
	2								
	1								

Fig. 3.9 Worksheet Data for Chap. 3: Practice Problem #2

Create an Excel spreadsheet with these data.

(a) Use Excel to the right of the table to find the sample size, mean, standard deviation, and standard error of the mean for these data. Label your answers, and use one decimal place for the mean, standard deviation, and standard error of the mean

(b) Enter the null hypothesis and the research hypothesis for this item on your spreadsheet.

(c) Use Excel's TINV function to find the 95% confidence interval about the mean for these data. Label your answers on your spreadsheet. Use one decimal place for the lower limit and the upper limit of the confidence interval.

(d) Enter the *result* of the test on your spreadsheet.
(e) Enter the *conclusion* of the test in plain English on your spreadsheet.
(f) Print your final spreadsheet so that it fits onto one page (if you need help remembering how to do this, see the objectives at the end of Chap. 2 in Sect. 2.4).
(g) Draw a picture of the confidence interval, including the reference value, onto your spreadsheet.
(h) Save the final spreadsheet as: ELDER3

3. The National Association of Social Workers (NASW) includes more than 132,000 social workers in the world as its members. NASW has chapters in all 50 states of the USA. The Web site includes a Professional Education and Training Center that specializes in a continuing education resource center for its members. The site also includes a Social Work Career center entitled: "Find a Job" which allows members to post their resume free of charge.

   Suppose that you have been asked to design an online survey that can be emailed to members of NASW who have visited this "Find a Job" site within the past 90 days. You are in the early stages of survey design, but you have decided that you do want to include the rating scale below as Item #16 in this online survey. You want to test your Excel skills on this type of survey, and so you have created the hypothetical data for this one item that are given in Fig.3.10.

NATIONAL ASSOCIATION OF SOCIAL WORKERS (NASW)

"Find a Job" Site in the Social Work Career Center

Item #16 "How helpful did you find this site in learning about job possibilities in the field of Social Work?"

1	2	3	4	5	6	7
Not Helpful						Very Helpful

Rating
5
6
2
3
4
7
5
6
7
7
6
4
5
3
5
6
7
6
5
6
4
3

Fig. 3.10 Worksheet Data for Chap. 3: Practice Problem #3

Create an Excel spreadsheet with these data.

(a) Use Excel to the right of the table to find the sample size, mean, standard deviation, and standard error of the mean for these data. Label your answers, and use two decimal places for the mean, standard deviation, and standard error of the mean

(b) Enter the null hypothesis and the research hypothesis for this item onto your spreadsheet.

(c) Use Excel's TINV function to find the 95% confidence interval about the mean for these data. Label your answers on your spreadsheet. Use two decimal places for the lower limit and the upper limit of the confidence interval.

(d) Enter the *result* of the test on your spreadsheet.
(e) Enter the *conclusion* of the test in plain English on your spreadsheet.
(f) Print your final spreadsheet so that it fits onto one page (if you need help remembering how to do this, see the objectives at the end of Chap. 2 in Sect. 2.4).
(g) Draw a picture of the confidence interval, including the reference value, onto your spreadsheet.
(h) Save the final spreadsheet as: social3

References

Black K. Business statistics: for contemporary decision making. 6th ed. Hoboken: John Wiley& Sons, Inc.; 2010.
Keller G. Statistics for management and economics. 8th ed. Mason: South-Western Cengage Learning; 2009.
McDaniel C, Gates R. Marketing research. 8th ed. Hoboken: John Wiley & Sons, Inc.; 2010.
Polit D F. Statistics and data analysis for nursing research. 2nd ed. Upper Saddle River: Pearson Education, Inc.; 2010.
Rosenthal J. Statistics and data interpretation for social work. New York: Springer Publishing Company, 2012.
Royse D. Research methods in social work. 6th ed. Belmont, CA: Cengage Learning; 2010.
Salkind N. Statistics for people who (think they) hate statistics. 2nd Excel 2007 ed. Los Angeles: Sage Publications; 2010.
Veney J E, Kros J F., Rosenthal D A. Statistics for health care professionals: working with Excel. San Francisco: Jossey-Bass; 2009.
Veney J E. Statistics for health policy and administration using Miocrosoft Excel. San Francisco: Jossey-Bass; 2003.
Weiers R. Introduction to business statistics. 7th ed. Mason: South-Western Cengage Learning; 2011.
Weinbach R. Statistics for social workers. 8th ed. Boston: Allyn & Bacon; 2010.
Zikmund W, Babin B. Exploring marketing research. 10th ed. Mason: South-Western Cengage Learning; 2010.

Chapter 4
One-Group t-Test for the Mean

In this chapter, you will learn how to use one of the most popular and most helpful statistical tests in social work research: the one-group t-test for the mean. One-group t-tests are used to determine whether there is a significant difference between a sample mean and a population mean.

The formula for the one-group t-test is as follows:

$$t = \frac{\bar{X} - \mu}{S_{\bar{X}}} \text{ where} \tag{4.1}$$

$$\text{s.e.} = S_{\bar{X}} = \frac{S}{\sqrt{n}} \tag{4.2}$$

This formula asks you to take the sample mean ($\bar{X}$) and subtract the population mean (μ) from it, and then divide the answer by the standard error of the sample mean (s.e.). The standard error of the sample mean equals the standard deviation divided by the square root of n (the sample size). If you want to learn more about this test, see Veney et al. (2009) and Schneider (2010).

Let's discuss the 7 STEPS of hypothesis testing using the one-group t-test so that you can understand how this test is used.

4.1 The 7 STEPS for Hypothesis-Testing Using the One-Group t-Test

Objective: To learn the 7 steps of hypothesis-testing using the one-group t-test

T.J. Quirk, S. Cummings, *Excel 2016 for Social Work Statistics*, Excel for Statistics,
DOI 10.1007/978-3-319-66221-3_4

Before you can try out your Excel skills on the one-group t-test, you need to learn the basic steps of hypothesis-testing for this statistical test. There are 7 steps in this process:

4.1.1 STEP 1: State the Null Hypothesis and the Research Hypothesis

Recall from Sect. 3.2.2 that the null hypothesis is what we accept as true unless we have compelling evidence that it is not true, which is generally a hypothesis of no difference between the sample mean and the population mean. The research hypothesis, on the other hand, is the alternative, i.e., a hypothesized difference between the sample mean and the population mean.

If you are using numerical scales in your survey, you need to remember that these hypotheses refer to the "middle" of the numerical scale. For example, if you are using 7-point scales with 1 = poor and 7 = excellent, these hypotheses would refer to the middle of these scales and would be:

Null hypothesis H_0: $\mu = 4$
Research hypothesis H_1: $\mu \neq 4$

As a second example, Royse (2010) discusses a Job Satisfaction Scale (JSS) that has been used with social service professionals. The rating scales for the JSS range from Very Dissatisfied (scored as 1), to Very Satisfied (scored as 11). Degree of Satisfaction is measured for 14 items on the instrument (e.g. Item #4 is: "Opportunities for promotion"). The hypotheses for testing each item on the JSS would be:

H_0 : $\mu = 6$
H_1 : $\mu \neq 6$

Note that these hypotheses are correct because there are five numbers below 6 (i.e., 1–5), and five numbers above 6 (i.e., 7–11).

4.1.2 STEP 2: Select the Appropriate Statistical Test

In this chapter we will be studying the one-group t-test, and so we will select that test.

4.1.3 STEP 3: Decide on a Decision Rule for the One-Group t-Test

(a) If the absolute value of t is less than the critical value of t , accept the null hypothesis.

(b) If the absolute value of t is greater than the critical value of t , reject the null hypothesis and accept the research hypothesis.

You are probably saying to yourself: "That sounds fine, but how do I find the absolute value of t?"

4.1.3.1 Finding the Absolute Value of a Number

To do that, we need another objective:

Objective: To find the absolute value of a number

If you took a basic algebra course in high school, you may remember the concept of "absolute value." In mathematical terms, the absolute value of any number is *always* that number expressed as a positive number.

For example, the absolute value of 2.35 is +2.35.

And the absolute value of minus 2.35 (i.e. −2.35) is also +2.35.

This becomes important when you are using the t-table in Appendix E of this book. We will discuss this table later when we get to Step 5 of the one-group t-test where we explain how to find the critical value of t using Appendix E.

4.1.4 STEP 4:Calculate the Formula for the One-Group t-Test

Objective: To learn how to use the formula for the one-group t-test

The formula for the one-group t-test is as follows:

$$t = \frac{\bar{X} - \mu}{S_{\bar{X}}} \text{ where} \tag{4.1}$$

$$\text{s.e.} = S_{\bar{X}} = \frac{S}{\sqrt{n}} \tag{4.2}$$

This formula makes the following assumptions about the data (Foster et al. 1998): (1) The data are independent of each other (i.e., each person or event receives only one score), (2) the *population* of the data is normally distributed, and (3) the data have a constant variance (note that the standard deviation is the square root of the variance).

To use this formula, you need to follow these steps:

1. Take the sample mean in your research study and subtract the population mean μ from it (remember that the population mean for a study involving numerical rating scales is the "middle" number in the scale).
2. Take your answer from the above step, and divide it by the standard error of the mean for your research study (remember that you learned how to find the standard error of the mean in Chap. 1; to find the standard error of the mean, just take the standard deviation of your research study and divide it by the square root of n , where n is the number of people or events in your research study).
3. The number you get after you complete the above step is the value for t that results when you use the formula stated above.

4.1.5 STEP 5: Find the Critical Value of t in the t-Table in Appendix E

Objective: To find the critical value of t in the t-table in Appendix E

Before we get into an explanation of what is meant by "the critical value of t," let's give you practice finding the critical value of t by using the t-table in Appendix E.

Keep your finger on Appendix E as we explain how you need to "read" that table.

Since the test in this chapter is called the "one-group t-test," you will use the first column on the left in Appendix E to find the critical value of t for your research study (note that this column is headed: "sample size n").

To find the critical value of t, you go down this first column until you find the sample size in your research study, and then you go to the right and read the critical value of t for that sample size in the critical t column in the table (note that *this is the column that you would use for both the one-group t-test and the 95% confidence interval about the mean*).

For example, if you have 27 people in your research study, the critical value of t is 2.056.

If you have 38 people in your research study, the critical value of t is 2.026.

If you have more than 40 people in your research study, the critical value of t is always 1.96.

Note that the "critical t column" in Appendix E represents the value of t that you need to obtain to be 95% confident that your results are "significant".

The critical value of t is the value that tells you whether or not you have found a "significant result" in your statistical test.

The t-table in Appendix E represents a series of "bell-shaped normal curves" (they are called bell-shaped because they look like the outline of the Liberty Bell that you can see in Philadelphia outside of Independence Hall).

The "middle" of these normal curves is treated as if it were zero point on the x-axis (the technical explanation of this fact is beyond the scope of this book, but any good statistics book (e.g. Zikmund and Babin 2010) will explain this concept to you if you are interested in learning more about it).

Thus, values of t that are to the right of this zero point are positive values that use a plus sign before them, and values of t that are to the left of this zero point are negative values that use a minus sign before them. Thus, some values of t are positive, and some are negative.

However, every statistics book that includes a t-table only reprints the *positive* side of the t-curves because the negative side is the mirror image of the positive side; this means that the negative side contains the exact same numbers as the positive side, but the negative numbers all have a minus sign in front of them.

Therefore, to use the t-table in Appendix E, you need to *take the absolute value of the t-value you found when you use the t-test formula* since the t-table in Appendix E only has the positive values for t.

Throughout this book, we assume that you want to be 95% confident in the results of your statistical tests. Therefore, the value for t in the t-table in Appendix E tells you whether or not the t-value you obtained when you used the formula for the one-group t-test is within the 95% interval of the t-curve range.

If the t-value you obtained when you used the formula for the one-group t-test is *inside* of the 95% confidence range, we say that the result you found is *not significant* (note that this is equivalent to *accepting the null hypothesis!)*.

If the t-value you found when you used the formula for the one-group t-test is *outside* of this 95% confidence range, we say that you have found a *significant result* that would be expected to occur less than 5% of the time (note that this is equivalent to *rejecting the null hypothesis and accepting the research hypothesis*).

4.1.6 STEP 6: State the Result of Your Statistical Test

There are two possible results when you use the one-group t-test, and only one of them can be accepted as "true."

Either: Since the absolute value of t that you found in the t-test formula is *less than the critical value of t* in Appendix E, you accept the null hypothesis.

Or: Since the absolute value of t that you found in the t-test formula is *greater than the critical value of t* in Appendix E, you reject the null hypothesis, and accept the research hypothesis.

4.1.7 STEP 7: State the Conclusion of Your Statistical Test in Plain English!

In practice, this is more difficult than it sounds because you are trying to summarize the result of your statistical test in simple English that is both concise and accurate so that someone who has never had a statistics course (such as your boss, perhaps) can understand the conclusion of your test. This is a difficult task, and we will give you lots of practice doing this last and most important step throughout this book.

If you have read this far, you are ready to sit down at your computer and perform the one-group t-test using Excel on some hypothetical data.

Let's give this a try.

4.2 One-Group t-Test for the Mean

The American College of Healthcare Executives (ACHE) is an international professional society of more than 40,000 healthcare professionals who work in a variety of healthcare organizations. ACHE is proud of its career development activities that are provided on its website. One of its most important career development activities is the posting of possible job-openings at healthcare organizations so that its members can be made aware of job-openings in the healthcare industry. Suppose that ACHE has asked its members who access its website to rate the helpfulness of its Career Services section in notifying members of job-openings in the healthcare industry, and you have been asked to analyze the resulting data. The data are based on visitors to the website who used the Career Services section. Suppose that Item #7 on the survey asked visitors to rate the helpfulness of the job-posting feature on a 10-point scale where 1 = poor and 10 = excellent.

The survey contains a number of items, but suppose a hypothetical Item #7 is the one in Fig. 4.1:

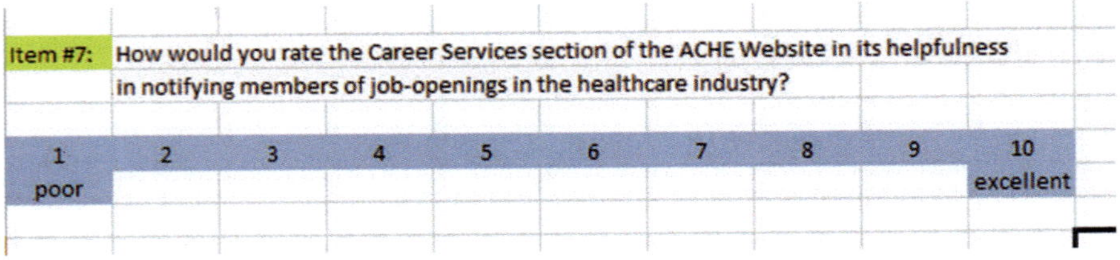

Fig. 4.1 Sample Survey Item for Item #7 of the ACHE Survey (Practical Example)

Suppose further, that you have decided to analyze the data from members using a one-group t-test.

Important note: You would need to use this test for each of the survey items separately.

Suppose that the hypothetical data for Item #7 of the ACHE Website were based on a sample size of 124 members who had a mean score on this item of 6.58 and a standard deviation on this item of 2.44.

Objective: To analyze the data for each question separately using a one-group t-test for each survey item.

Create an Excel spreadsheet with the following information:

B11: Null hypothesis:
B14: Research hypothesis:

Note: Remember that when you are using a rating scale item, both the null hypothesis and the research hypothesis refer to the "middle of the scale." For the 10-point scale in this example, the middle of the scale is 5.5 since five numbers are below 5.5 (i.e., 1–5) and five numbers are above 5.5 (i.e. 6–10). Therefore, the hypotheses for this rating scale item are:

$H_0: \quad \mu = 5.5$
$H_1: \quad \mu \neq 5.5$

B17: n
B20: mean
B23: STDEV
B26: s.e.
B29: critical t
B32: t-test
B36: Result:
B41: Conclusion:

Now, use Excel:

D17: enter the sample size
D20: enter the mean
D23: enter the STDEV (see Fig. 4.2)

Fig. 4.2 Basic Data Table for Item #7 of the ACHE Survey

Null hypothesis:		
Research hypothesis:		
n		124
mean		6.58
STDEV		2.44
s.e.		
critical t		
t-test		
Result:		
Conclusion:		

D26: compute the standard error using the formula in Chap. 1
D29: find the critical t value of t in the t-table in Appendix E

Now, enter the following formula in cell D32 to find the t-test result:

=(D20 − 5.5)/D26 (no spaces between symbols)

In Excel, this formula takes the sample mean (D20) and subtracts the population hypothesized mean of 5.5 from the sample mean, and THEN divides the answer by the standard error of the mean (D26). Note that you need to enter D20 − 5.5 with an open-parenthesis *before* D20 and a closed-parenthesis *after* 5.5 so that the *answer of 1.08 is THEN divided by the standard error of 0.22* to get the t-test result of 4.93.

Now, use two decimal places for both the s.e. and the t-test result (see Fig. 4.3).

Null hypothesis:		
Research hypothesis:		
n		124
mean		6.58
STDEV		2.44
s.e.		0.22
critical t		1.96
t-test		4.93
Result:		
Conclusion:		

Fig. 4.3 t-test Formula Result for Item #7 of the ACHE Survey

Now, write the following sentence in D36:D39 to summarize the result of the t-test:

D36: Since the absolute value of t of 4.93 is
D37: greater than the critical t of 1.96, we
D38: reject the null hypothesis and accept
D39: the research hypothesis.

Lastly, write the following sentence in D41:D44 to summarize the conclusion of the result for Item #7 of the ACHE Survey:

D41: Members rated the helpfulness of the Career
D42: Services section of the ACHE Website in its
D43: helpfulness in notifying members of job-openings
D44: in the healthcare industry as significantly positive.

Save your file as: career4C

Important note: *We have used the term "significantly positive" because the mean rating of 6.58 is on the positive side of the rating scale. We purposely have not used the term "significantly excellent" because people who speak English do not use that term because something is either excellent or it is not excellent. Therefore, "significantly positive" is a more correct use of the English language in this type of rating scale item.*

Important note: *You are probably wondering why we entered both the result and the conclusion in separate cells instead of in just one cell. This is because if you enter them in one cell, you will be very disappointed when you print out your final spreadsheet, because one of two things will happen that you will not like: (1) if you print the spreadsheet to fit onto only one page, the result and the conclusion will force the entire spreadsheet to be printed in such small font size that you will be unable to read it, or (2) if you do not print the final spreadsheet to fit onto one page, both the result and the conclusion will "dribble over" onto a second page instead of fitting the entire spread-sheet onto one page. In either case, your spread-sheet will not have a "professional look."*

Print the final spreadsheet so that it fits onto one page as given in Fig. 4.4. Enter the null hypothesis and the research hypothesis by hand on your spreadsheet

Null hypothesis:		μ	=	5.5
Research hypothesis:		μ	≠	5.5
n	124			
mean	6.58			
STDEV	2.44			
s.e.	0.22			
critical t	1.96			
t-test	4.93			
Result:		Since the absolute value of t of 4.93 is greater than the critical t of 1.96, we reject the null hypothesis and accept the research hypothesis.		
Conclusion:		Members rated the helpfulness of the Career Services section of the ACHE Website in its helpfulness in notifying members of job-openings in the healthcare indsustry as significantly positive.		

Fig. 4.4 Final Spreadsheet for Item #7 of the ACHE Survey

IMPORTANT NOTE: It is important for you to understand that "technically" the above conclusion in statistical terms should state:

"Members rated the helpfulness of the Career Services section of the ACHE Website in its helpfulness in notifying members of job-openings in the healthcare industry as positive, and this result was probably not obtained by chance."

However, throughout this book, we are using the term "significantly" in writing the conclusion of statistical tests to alert the reader that the result of the statistical test was probably not a chance finding, but instead of writing all of those words each time, we use the word "significantly" as a shorthand to the longer explanation. This makes it much easier for the reader to understand the conclusion when it is written "in plain English," instead of technical, statistical language.

4.3 Can You Use Either the 95% Confidence Interval About the Mean OR the One-Group t-Test When Testing Hypotheses?

You are probably asking yourself:

"It sounds like you could use *either* the 95% confidence interval about the mean *or* the one-group t-test to analyze the results of the types of problems described so far in this book? Is this a correct statement?"

The answer is a resounding: *"Yes!"*

Both the confidence interval about the mean and the one-group t-test are often used in research on the types of problems described so far in this book. *Both of these tests produce the same result and the same conclusion from the same data set!*

Both of these tests are explained in this book because some researchers prefer the confidence interval about the mean test, while others prefer the one-group t-test, and still others prefer to use both tests on the same data to make their results and conclusions clearer to the reader of their research reports. Since we do not know which of these tests your researcher prefers, we have explained both of them so that you are competent in the use of both tests in the analysis of statistical data.

Now, let's try your Excel skills on the one-group t-test on the three problems at the end of this chapter.

4.4 End-of-Chapter Practice Problems

1. Suppose that the Dean of the School of Social Work has asked you to analyze the data from a recent survey to MSW graduates from five years ago to obtain their feedback with their education in the School's MSW program. Suppose, further, the survey had 20 items in it, but that the Dean wants you to analyze the data this week for Item #20, and to analyze the data for the other 19 items over the next three weeks. You want to practice your Excels skills, and so you have created the hypothetical data for this question that are given in Fig. 4.5.

MSW SURVEY OF GRADUATES FROM FIVE YEARS AGO								
Item #20:	**How satisfied are you with the quality of social work education that you received in your MSW program?**							
1	**2**	**3**	**4**	**5**	**6**	**7**	**8**	**9**
very dissatisfied								**very satisfied**
		DATA						
		5						
		6						
		4						
		3						
		7						
		8						
		6						
		5						
		9						
		7						
		6						
		4						
		6						
		8						
		6						
		7						
		5						
		8						
		9						

Fig. 4.5 Worksheet Data for Chap. 4: Practice Problem #1

(a) Write the null hypothesis and the research hypothesis on your spreadsheet
(b) Use Excel to find the sample size, mean, standard deviation, and standard error of the mean to the right of the data set. Use number format (two decimal places) for the mean, standard deviation, and standard error of the mean.
(c) Enter the critical t from the t-table in Appendix E onto your spreadsheet, and label it.
(d) Use Excel to compute the t-value for these data (use two decimal places) and label it on your spreadsheet
(e) Type the result on your spreadsheet, and then type the conclusion in plain English on your spreadsheet
(f) Save the file as: survey23

2. The Department of Managed Health Care in the State of California (USA) has adopted a number of regulations to ensure that managed care enrollees have access to healthcare services in a timely manner. One of these regulations requires that health care plans show that their provider networks are sufficiently large to ensure that enrollees be offered an appointment with a primary care

provider within 10 business days of such a request. Suppose that you are an intern for a health insurer and that you have been asked to determine whether or not your company is in compliance with this regulation. Hypothetical data on a random sample of patients insured with your company are presented in Fig. 4.6:

NUMBER OF DAYS FROM REQUEST FOR AN APPOINTMENT TO APPOINTMENT DATE

PATIENT	NO. OF APPOINTMENT DAYS
1	7
2	18
3	12
4	16
5	19
6	21
7	8
8	6
9	4
10	15
11	16
12	18
13	17
14	16
15	12
16	9
17	11
18	14
19	13

Fig. 4.6 Worksheet Data for Chap. 4: Practice Problem #2

(a) *On your Excel spreadsheet*, write the null hypothesis and the research hypothesis for these data.
(b) Use Excel to find the sample size, mean, standard deviation, and standard error of the mean for these data (two decimal places for the mean, standard deviation, and standard error of the mean).
(c) Use Excel to perform a one-group t-test on these data (two decimal places).
(d) On your printout, type the critical value of t given in your t-table in Appendix E.
(e) On your spreadsheet, type the result of the t-test.
(f) On your spreadsheet, type the conclusion of your study in plain English.
(g) save the file as: DISCHARGE3

3. Suppose that you have been asked to design a survey that can be administered to recent clients who have completed an alcohol treatment program in your facility. You are in the early stages of design of this survey, but you have decided that Item #24 of the survey should ask clients how likely they would be to recommend this program to a friend who needed similar help. You want to test your Excel skills, so you have created the hypothetical data for this item that is given in Fig. 4.7.

ALCOHOL TREATMENT FACILITY						
	Client Satisfaction Survey					
Item #24:	**If a friend needed similar help with an alcohol treatment facility, how likely would you be to recommend this program to this friend?"**					
1	**2**	**3**	**4**	**5**	**6**	**7**
Very Unlikely						**Very Likely**
		DATA				
		5				
		4				
		5				
		3				
		7				
		5				
		4				
		6				
		5				
		2				
		3				
		5				
		4				
		6				
		4				
		5				
		6				
		4				

Fig. 4.7 Worksheet Data for Chap. 4: Practice problem #3

(a) Write the null hypothesis and the research hypothesis on your spreadsheet
(b) Use Excel to find the sample size, mean, standard deviation, and standard error of the mean to the right of the data set. Use number format (two decimal places) for the mean, standard deviation, and standard error of the mean.
(c) Enter the critical t from the t-table in Appendix E onto your spreadsheet, and label it.
(d) Use Excel to compute the t-value for these data (use two decimal places) and label it on your spreadsheet
(e) Type the result on your spreadsheet, and then type the conclusion in plain English on your spreadsheet
(f) Save the file as: ALCOHOL3

References

Foster D, Stine R, Waterman R. Basic business statistics: a casebook. New York: Springer-Verlag; 1998.

Royse D. Research methods in social work. 6th ed. Belmont CA: Cengage Learning; 2010.

Schneider R. Basic statistics for social workers. Revised ed. Lanham MD: University Press of America; 2010.

Veney J E, Kros J F, Rosenthal D A. Statistics for health care professionals: working with Excel. 2nd ed. San Francisco: Jossey-Bass; 2009.

Zikmund W, Babin B. Exploring marketing research. 10th ed. Mason: South-Western Cengage Learning; 2010.

Chapter 5
Two-Group t-Test of the Difference of the Means for Independent Groups

Up until now in this book, you have been dealing with the situation in which you have had only one group of people or events in your research study and only one measurement "number" on each of these people or events. We will now change gears and deal with the situation in which you are measuring two groups instead of only one group.

Whenever you have two completely different groups of people or events (i.e., no one person or event is in both groups, but every person or event is measured on only one variable to produce one "number" for each person or event), we say that the two groups are "independent of one another." This chapter deals with just that situation.

Two assumptions underly the two-group t-test (Wheater and Cook 2000): (1) both groups are sampled from a normal population, and (2) the variances of the two populations are approximately equal. Note that the standard deviation is merely the square root of the variance. (There are different formulas to use when each person or event is measured twice to create two groups of data, and this situation is called "dependent," but those formulas are beyond the scope of this book.) This book only deals with two groups that are independent of one another so that no person or event is in both groups of data.

When you test for the difference between the means for two groups, it is important to remember that there are two different formulas that you need to use depending on the sample sizes of the two groups:

(1) Use Formula #1 in this chapter when both of the groups have a sample size greater than 30, and
(2) Use Formula #2 in this chapter when either one group, or both groups, have a sample size less than 30.

We will illustrate both of these situations in this chapter.

But, first, we need to understand the steps involved in hypothesis-testing when two groups are involved before we dive into the formulas for these tests.

T.J. Quirk, S. Cummings, *Excel 2016 for Social Work Statistics*, Excel for Statistics,
DOI 10.1007/978-3-319-66221-3_5

5.1 The 9 STEPS for Hypothesis-Testing Using the Two-Group t-Test

Objective: To learn the 9 steps of hypothesis-testing using two groups of people or events and the two-group t-test

You will see that these steps parallel the steps used in the previous chapter that dealt with the one-group t-test, but there are some important differences between the steps that you need to understand clearly before we dive into the formulas for the two-group t-test.

5.1.1 STEP 1: Name One Group, Group 1, and the Other Group, Group 2

The formulas used in this chapter will use the numbers 1 and 2 to distinguish between the two groups. If you define which group is Group 1 and which group is Group 2, you can use these numbers in your computations without having to write out the names of the groups.

For example, if you were testing entering college freshmen who said they wanted to major in social work to see if there were gender differences in their SAT-Math scores as high school seniors, you could call the groups: "Freshmen Males" and "Freshmen Females," but this would require you to write out the words "Freshmen Males" and "Freshmen Females" whenever you wanted to refer to one of these groups. If you call the "Freshmen Males" group, Group 1, and the "Freshmen Females" group, Group 2, this makes it much easier to refer to the groups because it saves writing time.

Note, also, that it is completely arbitrary which group you name Group 1, and which Group you name Group 2. You will achieve the same result and the same conclusion from the formulas however you decide to define these two groups.

5.1.2 STEP 2: Create a Table That Summarizes the Sample Size, Mean Score, and Standard Deviation of Each Group

This step makes it easier for you to make sure that you are using the correct numbers in the formulas for the two-group t-test. If you get the numbers "mixed-up," your entire formula work will be incorrect and you will botch the problem terribly.

For example, suppose that you collected data on entering freshmen who said that they planned to major in social work (BSW) and found that the Freshmen Males group had 57 men in it and their SAT-Math scores averaged 610 with a standard deviation of 120, while the Freshmen Females group had 46 females in it and their SAT-Math scores averaged 640 with a standard deviation of 110.

The formulas for analyzing these data to determine if there was a significant different in the average SAT-Math score for Freshmen Males *versus* Freshmen Females require you to use six numbers correctly: the sample size, the mean, and the standard deviation of each of the two groups. All six of these numbers must be used correctly in the formulas if you are to analyze the data correctly.

If you create a table to summarize these data, a good example of the table, using both Step 1 and Step 2, would be the data presented in Fig. 5.1:

Fig. 5.1 Basic Table Format for the Two-Group t-Test

A	B	C	D	E	F
	Group	n	Mean	STDEV	
	1 (name it)				
	2 (name it)				

If you decide to name Group 1 the Freshmen Males group and Group 2 the Freshmen Females group, the following table would place the six numbers from your research study into the proper cells of the table as in Fig. 5.2:

	A	B	C	D	E	F
1						
2						
3		Group	n	Mean	STDEV	
4		1 Freshmen Males SAT-Math scores	57	610	120	
5		2 Freshmen Females SAT-Math scores	46	640	110	
6						

Fig. 5.2 Results of Entering the Data Needed for the Two-Group t-Test

You can now use the formulas for the two-group t-test with more confidence that the six numbers will be placed in the proper place in the formulas.

Note that you could just as easily name Group 1 the Freshmen Females group and Group 2 the Freshmen Males group; it makes no difference how you decide to name the two groups; this decision is up to you and you will get the same result from your statistical test no matter which decision you make.

5.1.3 STEP 3: State the Null Hypothesis and the Research Hypothesis for the Two-Group t-Test

If you have completed Step 1 above, this step is very easy because the null hypothesis and the research hypothesis will always be stated in the same way for the two-group t-test. The null hypothesis states that the population means of the two groups are equal, while the research hypothesis states that the population means of the two groups are not equal. In notation format, this becomes:

$H_0: \quad \mu_1 = \mu_2$
$H_1: \quad \mu_1 \neq \mu_2$

You can now see that this notation is much simpler than having to write out the names of the two groups in all of your formulas.

5.1.4 STEP 4: Select the Appropriate Statistical Test

Since this chapter deals with the situation in which you have two groups but only one measurement on each person or event in each group, we will use the two-group t-test throughout this chapter.

5.1.5 STEP 5: Decide on a Decision Rule for the Two-Group t-Test

The decision rule is exactly the same as what it was in the previous chapter (see Sect. 4.1.3) when we dealt with the one-group t-test.

(a) If the absolute value of t is less than the critical value of t, accept the null hypothesis.
(b) If the absolute value of t is greater than the critical value of t, reject the null hypothesis and accept the research hypothesis.

Since you learned how to find the absolute value of t in the previous chapter (see Sect. 4.1.3.1), you can use that knowledge in this chapter.

5.1.6 STEP 6: Calculate the Formula for the Two-Group t-Test

Since we are using two different formulas in this chapter for the two-group t-test depending on the sample size in the two groups, we will explain how to use those formulas later in this chapter.

5.1.7 STEP 7: Find the Critical Value of t in the t-Table in Appendix E

In the previous chapter where we were dealing with the one-group t-test, you found the critical value of t in the t-table in Appendix E by finding the sample size for the one group in the first column of the table, and then reading the critical value of t across from it on the right in the "critical t column" in the table (see Sect. 4.1.5). This process is fairly simple once you have had some practice in doing this step.

However, for the two-group t-test, the procedure for finding the critical value of t is more complicated because you have two different groups in your study, and they often have different sample sizes in each group.

To use Appendix E correctly in this chapter, you need to learn how to find the "degrees of freedom" for your study. We will discuss that process now.

5.1.7.1 Find the Degrees of Freedom (df) for the Two-Group t-Test

Objective: To find the degrees of freedom for the two-group t-test and to use it to find the critical value of t in the t-table in Appendix E

The mathematical explanation of "degrees of freedom" is beyond the scope of this book, but you can find out more about this concept by reading any good statistics book (e.g. Keller 2009 or Bowers 2008). For our purposes, you can easily understand how to find degrees of freedom and to use it to find the critical value of t in Appendix E. The formula for the degrees of freedom (df) is:

$$\text{degrees of freedom} = \text{df} = n_1 + n_2 - 2 \quad (5.1)$$

In other words, you add the sample size for Group 1 to the sample size for Group 2 and then subtract 2 from this total to get the number of degrees of freedom to use in Appendix E.

Take a look at Appendix E.

Instead of using the first column as we did in the one-group t-test that is based on the sample size, n, of one group, we need to use the second-column of this table (df) to find the critical value of t for the two-group t-test.

For example, if you had 13 people in Group 1 and 17 people in Group 2, the degrees of freedom would be: 13 + 17 − 2 = 28, and the critical value of t would be 2.048 *since you look down the second column which contains the degrees of freedom* until you come to the number 28, and then read 2.048 in the "critical t column" in the table to find the critical value of t when df = 28.

As a second example, if you had 52 people in Group 1 and 57 people in Group 2, the degrees of freedom would be: 52 + 57 − 2 = 107. When you go down the second column in Appendix E for the degrees of freedom, you find that *once you go beyond the degrees of freedom equal to 39, the critical value of t is always 1.96*, and that is the value you would use for the critical t with this example.

5.1.8 STEP 8: State the Result of Your Statistical Test

The result follows the exact same result format that you found for the one-group t-test in the previous chapter (see Sect. 4.1.6):

Either: Since the absolute value of t that you found in the t-test formula is *less than the critical value of t* in Appendix E, you accept the null hypothesis.

Or: Since the absolute value of t that you found in the t-test formula is *greater than the critical value of t* in Appendix E, you reject the null hypothesis and accept the research hypothesis.

5.1.9 STEP 9: State the Conclusion of Your Statistical Test in Plain English!

Writing the conclusion for the two-group t-test is more difficult than writing the conclusion for the one-group t-test because you have to decide what the difference was between the two groups.

When you accept the null hypothesis, the conclusion is simple to write: "There is no difference between the two groups in the variable that was measured."

But when you reject the null hypothesis and accept the research hypothesis, you need to be careful about writing the conclusion so that it is both accurate and concise.

Let's give you some practice in writing the conclusion of a two-group t-test.

5.1.9.1 Writing the Conclusion of the Two-Group t-Test When You Accept the Null Hypothesis

Objective: To write the conclusion of the two-group t-test when you have accepted the null hypothesis.

The American College of Healthcare Executives (ACHE) is an international professional organization with more than 40,000 members. ACHE's most important educational program is an annual Congress on Healthcare Leadership which typically has more than 4,000 participants. Suppose you have been asked to design a survey that can be emailed to participants after the Congress has ended to determine the attitude of participants toward the many activities of the Congress. One key item that you are sure that you want to include is an item asking participants if they would recommend attending next year's Congress to their colleagues. Item #10 of this survey is given in Fig. 5.3.

Item #10: **"How likely are you to recommend to colleagues that they attend next year's ACHE Congress on Healthcare Leadership?**

1	2	3	4	5	6	7	8	9	10
very unlikely									very likely

Fig. 5.3 ACHE Congress Evaluation Survey Item #10

Suppose further, that you have decided to analyze the data from the Survey comparing the attitudes of men who attended the Congress to those of women who attended the Congress by using the two-group t-test.

Important note: You would need to use this test for each of the Survey items separately.

Suppose that the hypothetical data for Item #10 was based on a sample size of 124 Males who had a mean score on this item of 6.58 and a standard deviation on this item of 2.44. Suppose that you also had data from 86 Females who had a mean score of 6.45 with a standard deviation of 1.86.

We will explain later in this chapter how to produce the results of the two-group t-test using its formulas, but, for now, let's "cut to the chase" and create a table for these data (see Fig. 5.4):

Fig. 5.4 Worksheet Data for Item #10 for Accepting the Null Hypothesis

Group	n	Mean	STDEV
1 Males	124	6.58	2.44
2 Females	86	6.45	1.86

degrees of freedom:	208
critical t:	1.96 (in Appendix E)
t-test formula:	0.44 (when you use your calculator!)
Result:	Since the absolute value of 0.44 is less than the critical t of 1.96, we accept the null hypothesis.
Conclusion:	There was no difference between Males and Females in their likelihood of recommending that colleagues attend next year's Congress.

Now, let's see what happens when you reject the null hypothesis (H_0) and accept the research hypothesis (H_1).

5.1.9.2 Writing the Conclusion of the Two-Group t-Test When You Reject the Null Hypothesis and Accept the Research Hypothesis

> Objective: To write the conclusion of the two-group t-test when you have rejected the null hypothesis and accepted the research hypothesis

Let's continue with this same example, but with the result that we reject the null hypothesis and accept the research hypothesis.

Let's assume that this time you have data on 85 Males and their mean score on Item #10 was 7.26 with a standard deviation of 2.35. Let's further suppose that you also have data on 48 Females and their mean score on this question was 4.37 with a standard deviation of 3.26. Let's call Males, Group 1, and Females, Group 2.

Without going into the details of the formulas for the two-group t-test, these data in a table would produce the following result and conclusion based on Fig. 5.5:

	A	B	C	D	E
1					
2					
3		Group	n	Mean	STDEV
4		1 Males	85	7.26	2.35
5		2 Females	48	4.37	3.26
6					

Fig. 5.5 Worksheet Data for Item #10 for Obtaining a Significant Difference between Males and Females

Null Hypothesis: $\mu_1 = \mu_2$
Research Hypothesis: $\mu_1 \neq \mu_2$
degrees of freedom: 131
critical t: 1.96 (in Appendix E)
t-test formula: 5.40 (when you use your calculator!)
Result: Since the absolute value of 5.40 is greater than the critical t of 1.96, we reject the null hypothesis and accept the research hypothesis.

Now, you need to write a conclusion comparing Males and Females on their likelihood of recommending to colleagues that they attend next year's Congress using the following rule:

Rule: To summarize the conclusion of the two-group t-test, just compare the means of the two groups, and be sure to use the word "significantly" in your conclusion if you rejected the null hypothesis and accepted the research hypothesis.

A good way to prepare to write the conclusion of the two-group t-test when you are using a rating scale is to place the mean scores of the two groups on a drawing of the scale so that you can visualize the difference between the mean scores. For example, using our ACHE Congress example from above, you would draw this "picture" of the scale in Fig. 5.6:

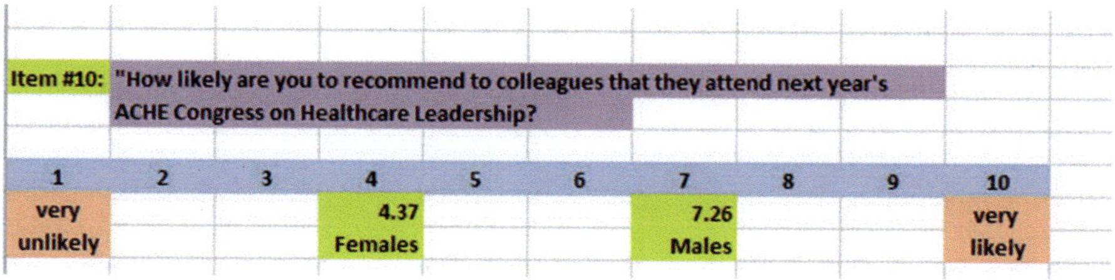

Fig. 5.6 Example of Drawing a "Picture" of the Means of the Two Groups on the Rating Scale

This drawing tells you visually that Males had a higher average rating than Females on Item #10 (7.26 vs. 4.37). *And, since you rejected the null hypothesis and accepted the research hypothesis, you know that you have found a significant difference between the two mean scores.*

So, our conclusion needs to contain the following key words:

- Males
- Females
- likelihood of recommending that colleagues attend next year's Congress
- significantly
- more likely or less likely
- *either* (7.26 vs. 4.37) *or* (4.37 vs. 7.26)

We can use these key words to write either of two conclusions, which are *logically identical*:

Either: Males were significantly more likely than Females to recommend that their colleagues attend next year's Congress (7.26 vs. 4.37).

Or: Females were significantly less likely than Males to recommend that their colleagues attend next year's Congress (4.37 vs. 7.26).

Both of these conclusions are accurate, so you can decide which one you want to write. It is your choice.

Also, note that the mean scores in parentheses at the end of these conclusions must match the sequence of the two groups in your conclusion. For example, if you say that: "Males were significantly more likely than Females," the end of this conclusion should be: (7.26 vs. 4.37) since you mentioned Males first, and Females second.

Alternately, if you wrote that: "Females were significantly less likely than Males," the end of this conclusion should be: (4.37 vs. 7.26) since you mentioned Females first, and Males second.

Putting the two mean scores at the end of your conclusion saves the reader from having to turn back to the table in your research report to find these mean scores to see how far apart they were.

Now, let's discuss FORMULA #1 that deals with the situation in which both groups have a sample size greater than 30.

Objective: To use FORMULA #1 for the two-group t-test when both groups have a sample size greater than 30

5.2 Formula #1: Both Groups Have a Sample Size Greater Than 30

The first formula we will discuss will be used when you have two groups with a sample size greater than 30 in each group and one measurement on each member in each group. This formula for the two-group t-test is:

$$t = \frac{\bar{X}_1 - \bar{X}_2}{S_{\bar{X}_1 - \bar{X}_2}} \tag{5.2}$$

$$\text{where } S_{\bar{X}_1 - \bar{X}_2} = \sqrt{\frac{{S_1}^2}{n_1} + \frac{{S_2}^2}{n_2}} \tag{5.3}$$

$$\text{and where degrees of freedom} = df = n_1 + n_2 - 2 \tag{5.1}$$

This formula looks daunting when you first see it, but let's explain some of the parts of this formula:

We have explained the concept of "degrees of freedom" earlier in this chapter, and so you should be able to find the degrees of freedom needed for this formula in order to find the critical value of t in Appendix E.

In the previous chapter, *the formula for the one-group t-test was the following*:

$$t = \frac{\bar{X} - \mu}{S_{\bar{X}}} \tag{4.1}$$

$$\text{where s.e.} = S_{\bar{X}} = \frac{S}{\sqrt{n}} \tag{4.2}$$

For the one-group t-test, you found the mean score and subtracted the population mean from it, and then divided the result by the standard error of the mean (s.e.) to get the result of the t-test. You then compared the t-test result to the critical value of t to see if you either accepted the null hypothesis, or rejected the null hypothesis and accepted the research hypothesis.

The two-group t-test requires a different formula because you have two groups, each with a mean score on some variable. You are trying to determine whether to accept the null hypothesis that the *population means of the two groups are equal* (in other words, there is no difference statistically between these two means), or whether the difference between the means of the two groups is "sufficiently large" that you would accept *that there is a significant difference* in the mean scores of the two groups.

The numerator of the two-group t-test asks you to find the difference between the means of the two groups:

$$\bar{X}_1 - \bar{X}_2 \quad (5.4)$$

The next step in the formula for the two-group t-test is to divide the answer you get when you subtract the two means by the standard error of the difference of the two means, and *this is a different standard error of the mean than the one you found for the one-group t-test because there are two means in the two-group t-test.*

The standard error of the mean when you have two groups is called the "standard error of the difference of the means." This formula looks less scary when you break it down into four steps:

1. Square the standard deviation of Group 1, and divide this result by the sample size for Group 1 (n_1).
2. Square the standard deviation of Group 2, and divide this result by the sample size for Group 2 (n_2).
3. Add the results of the above two steps to get a total score.
4. *Take the square root of this total score* to find the standard error of the difference of the means between the two groups, $S_{\bar{X}_1 - \bar{X}_2} = \sqrt{\frac{{S_1}^2}{n_1} + \frac{{S_2}^2}{n_2}}$

This last step is the one that gives students the most difficulty when they are finding this standard error using their calculator, because they are in such a hurry to get to the answer that they forget to carry the square root sign down to the last step, and thus get a larger number than they should for the standard error.

5.2.1 An Example of Formula #1 for the Two-Group t-Test

Now, let's use Formula #1 in a situation in which both groups have a sample size greater than 30.

Suppose that a university that offered a Master's degree in Social Work (MSW) wanted to obtain feedback from students at the end of a course in Managing Human Resources from the previous semester to determine if there was a gender difference in the students' opinions of the course. Item #12 of the Course Evaluation Form asked the graduate students for their overall rating of the quality of the course using a 100-point scale. This rating item is given in Fig. 5.7.

Item #12:	**Overall, how would you rate the quality of the Managing Human Resources course?**									
0	**10**	**20**	**30**	**40**	**50**	**60**	**70**	**80**	**90**	**100**
poor										**Excellent**

Fig. 5.7 Example of Item #12 of the Course Evaluation Form (Practical Example)

Suppose you collect these evaluation forms and determine (using your new Excel skills) that the 52 Males in Group 1 had a mean score of 55 with a standard deviation of 7, while the 57 Females in Group 2 had a mean score of 64 with a standard deviation of 13 on Item #12.

Note that the two-group t-test does not require that both groups have the same sample size. This is another way of saying that the two-group t-test is "robust" (a fancy term that statisticians like to use).

Your data then produce the following table in Fig. 5.8:

Fig. 5.8 Worksheet Data for item #12 for Managing Human Resources

	A	B	C	D	E	F
1						
2						
3		**Group**	**n**	**Mean**	**STDEV**	
4		**1 Males**	**52**	**55**	**7**	
5		**2 Females**	**57**	**64**	**13**	
6						

Create an Excel spreadsheet, and enter the following information:

B3: Group
B4: 1 Males
B5: 2 Females
C3: n
D3: Mean
E3: STDEV
C4: 52
D4: 55
E4: 7
C5: 57
D5: 64
E5: 13

Now, widen column B so that it is twice as wide as column A, and center the six numbers and their labels in your table (see Fig. 5.9)

Group	n	Mean	STDEV
1 Males	52	55	7
2 Females	57	64	13

Fig. 5.9 Results of Widening Column B and Centering the Numbers in the Cells

B8: Null hypothesis:
B10: Research hypothesis:

Since both groups have a sample size greater than 30, you need to use Formula #1 for the t-test for the difference of the means of the two groups.

Let's "break this formula down into pieces" to reduce the chance of making a mistake by entering the following information into the cells below.

B13: STDEV1 squared/n1 (note that you square the standard deviation of Group 1, and then divide the result by the sample size of Group 1)
B16: STDEV2 squared/n2
B19: D13 + D16
B22: s.e.
B25: critical t
B28: t-test
B31: Result:
B36: Conclusion: (see Fig. 5.10)

Fig. 5.10 Formula Labels for the Two-group t-test

Group	n	Mean	STDEV
1 Males	52	55	7
2 Females	57	64	13
Null hypothesis:			
Research hypothesis:			
STDEV1 squared / n1			
STDEV2 squared / n2			
D13+D16			
s.e.			
critical t			
t-test			
Result:			
Conclusion:			

You now need to compute the values of the above formulas in the following cells:

D13: the result of the formula needed to compute cell B13 (use two decimals)
D16: the result of the formula needed to compute cell B16 (use two decimals)
D19: the result of the formula needed to compute cell B19 (use two decimals)
D22: =SQRT(D19) (use two decimals)

This formula should give you a standard error (s.e.) of 1.98.

D25: 1.96

(Since df = n1 + n2 − 2, this gives df = 109 − 2 = 107, and the critical t is, therefore, 1.96 in Appendix E.)

D28: =(D4–D5)/D22 (use 2 decimals; no spaces between symbols)

This formula should give you a value for the t-test of: −4.55.

Next, check to see if you have rounded off all figures in D13:D28 to two decimal places (see Fig. 5.11).

Fig. 5.11 Results of the t-test Formula for Comparisons of Males vs. Females

Group	n	Mean	STDEV
1 Males	52	55	7
2 Females	57	64	13
Null hypothesis:			
Research hypothesis:			
STDEV1 squared / n1		0.94	
STDEV2 squared / n2		2.96	
D13+D16		3.91	
s.e.		1.98	
critical t		1.96	
t-test		- 4.55	
Result:			
Conclusion:			

Now, write the following sentence in D31 to D34 to summarize the result of the study:

D31: Since the absolute value of −4.55
D32: is greater than the critical t of
D33: 1.96, we reject the null hypothesis
D34: and accept the research hypothesis.

Finally, write the following sentence in D36 to D39 to summarize the conclusion of the study in plain English:

D36: Overall, Females rated the quality of the
D37: Managing Human Resources course
D38: this past term as significantly higher
D39: quality than Males (64 vs. 55).

Save your file as: EVAL12

Important note: You are probably wondering why we entered both the result and the conclusion in separate cells instead of in just one cell. This is because if you enter them in one cell, you will be very disappointed when you print out your final spreadsheet, because one of two things will happen that you will not like: (1) if you print the spreadsheet to fit onto only one page, the result and the conclusion will force the entire spreadsheet to be printed in such small font size that you will be unable to read it, or (2) if you do not print the final spreadsheet to fit onto one page, both the result and the conclusion will "dribble over" onto a second page instead of fitting the entire spreadsheet onto one page. In either case, your spreadsheet will not have a "professional look."

Print this file so that it fits onto one page, and write by hand the null hypothesis and the research hypothesis on your printout.

The final spreadsheet appears in Fig. 5.12.

Group	n	Mean	STDEV
1 Males	52	55	7
2 Females	57	64	13
Null hypothesis:	μ_1	=	μ_2
Research hypothesis:	μ_1	≠	μ_2
STDEV1 squared / n1		0.94	
STDEV2 squared / n2		2.96	
D13 + D16		3.91	
s.e.		1.98	
critical t		1.96	
t-test		-4.55	
Result:		Since the absolute value of − 4.55 is greater than the critical t of 1.96 we reject the null hypothesis and accept the research hypothesis.	
Conclusion:		Overall, Females rated the quality of the Managing Human Resources course this past term as significantly higher quality than Males (64 vs. 55).	

Fig. 5.12 Final Worksheet for Item #12 Comparing Males vs. Females

Now, let's use the second formula for the two-group t-test which we use whenever either one group, or both groups, have a sample size less than 30.

> Objective: To use Formula #2 for the two-group t-test when one or both groups have a sample size less than 30

Now, let's look at the case when one or both groups have a sample size less than 30.

5.3 Formula #2: One or Both Groups Have a Sample Size Less Than 30

We would use Formula #2 when the underlying population standard deviations are unknown, but are presumed to be equal.

Suppose that a healthcare administrator at a multi-institutional healthcare center wanted to determine the average number of days it took to transfer patients from two of its health care facilities to long-term care facilities after the patients were ready for discharge. Suppose, further, that the administrator asks you to take a random sample of transfer patients from both FACILITY A and FACILITY B over the past three months. You decide to try out your new Excel skills on a small sample of this type of patient on the hypothetical data given in Fig. 5.13:

DELAY IN TRANSFER COMPARISON OF TWO HEALTHCARE FACILITIES

FACILITY A	FACILITY B
9	8
21	21
10	16
12	18
15	13
11	20
13	16
9	18
11	15
12	17
14	19
13	20
10	21
15	19
17	18
11	16
9	17
10	15
11	13
	15
	16

Fig. 5.13 Worksheet Data for Delay in Transfer Comparisons (Practical Example)

Let's re-name FACILITY A Group 1, and re-name FACILITY B Group 2.

Null hypothesis: $\mu_1 = \mu_2$
Research hypothesis: $\mu_1 \neq \mu_2$

Note: Since both groups have a sample size less than 30, you need to use Formula #2 in the following steps:

Create an Excel spreadsheet, and enter the following information:

B2: DELAY IN TRANSFER COMPARISON OF TWO HEALTHCARE FACILITIES
B4: FACILITY A
C4: FACILITY B
B5: 9
B23: 11
C5: 8
C25: 16

Now, enter the other figures into this table. Be sure to double-check all of your figures. If you have only one incorrect figure, you will not be able to obtain the correct answer to this problem.

Now, widen columns B and C so that all of the information fits inside the cells. To do this, click on both letters B and C at the top of these columns on your spreadsheet to highlight all of the cells in columns B and C. Then, move the mouse pointer to the right end of the B cell until you get a "cross" sign; then, click on this cross sign and drag the sign to the right until you can read all of the words on your screen. Then, stop clicking! Both Column B and Column C should now be the same width.

Next, center all information in the table except the top title by using the following steps:

Left-click your mouse and highlight cells B4:C25. Then, click on the bottom line, second from the left icon, under "Alignment" at the top-center of Home. All of the information in the table should now be in the center of each cell.

E5: Null hypothesis:
E7: Research hypothesis:
E9: Group
E10: 1 FACILITY A
E11: 2 FACILITY B
F9: n
G9: Mean
H9: STDEV

Your spreadsheet should now look like Fig. 5.14.

DELAY IN TRANSFER COMPARISON OF TWO HEALTHCARE FACILITIES

FACILITY A	FACILITY B
9	8
21	21
10	16
12	18
15	13
11	20
13	16
9	18
11	15
12	17
14	19
13	20
10	21
15	19
17	18
11	16
9	17
10	15
11	13
	15
	16

Null hypothesis:

Research hypothesis:

Group	n	Mean	STDEV
1 FACILITY A			
2 FACILITY B			

Fig. 5.14 Worksheet Data for Hypothesis Testing

Now you need to use your Excel skills from Chap. 1 to fill in the sample sizes (n), the means, and the standard deviations (STDEV) in the Table in cells F10:H11. Be sure to double-check your work or you will not be able to obtain the correct answer to this problem if you have only one incorrect figure! Round off the means and standard deviations to zero decimal places and center these six figures within their cells.

Since both groups have a sample size less than 30, you need to use Formula #2 for the t-test for the difference of the means of two independent samples.

Formula #2 for the two-group t-test is the following:

$$t = \frac{\bar{X}_1 - \bar{X}_2}{S_{\bar{X}_1 - \bar{X}_2}} \tag{5.1}$$

$$\text{where } S_{\bar{X}_1 - \bar{X}_2} = \sqrt{\frac{(n_1 - 1)S_1{}^2 + (n_2 - 1)S_2{}^2}{n_1 + n_2 - 2}\left(\frac{1}{n_1} + \frac{1}{n_2}\right)} \tag{5.5}$$

$$\text{and where degrees of freedom} = df = n_1 + n_2 - 2 \tag{5.6}$$

This formula is complicated, and so it will reduce your chance of making a mistake in writing it if you "break it down into pieces" instead of trying to write the formula as one cell entry.

Now, enter these words on your spreadsheet:

E14: (n1 − 1) × STDEV1 squared
E16: (n2 − 1) × STDEV2 squared
E18: $n_1 + n_2 - 2$
E20: $1/n_1 + 1/n_2$
E23: s.e.
E26: critical t
E29: t-test
B32: Result:
B36: Conclusion: (see Fig. 5.15)

DELAY IN TRANSFER COMPARISON OF TWO HEALTHCARE FACILITIES

FACILITY A	FACILITY B
9	8
21	21
10	16
12	18
15	13
11	20
13	16
9	18
11	15
12	17
14	19
13	20
10	21
15	19
17	18
11	16
9	17
10	15
11	13
	15
	16

Null hypothesis:

Research hypothesis:

Group	n	Mean	STDEV
1 FACILITY A	19	12	3
2 FACILITY B	21	17	3

(n-1) x STDEV1 squared

(n2 - 1) x STDEV2 squared

n1 + n2 – 2

1/n1 + 1/n2

s.e.

critical t

t-test

Result:

Conclusion:

Fig. 5.15 Formula Labels for the Two-group t-test

You now need to use your Excel skills to compute the values of the above formulas in the following cells:

H14: the result of the formula needed to compute cell E14 (use two decimals)
H16: the result of the formula needed to compute cell E16 (use two decimals)
H18: the result of the formula needed to compute cell E18
H20: the result of the formula needed to compute cell E20 (use two decimals)
H23: =SQRT(((H14 + H16)/H18)*H20) (no spaces between symbols)

Note the three open-parentheses after SQRT, and the three closed parentheses on the right side of this formula. You need three open parentheses and three closed parentheses in this formula or the formula will not work correctly.

The above formula gives a standard error of the difference of the means equal to 0.97 (two decimals) in cell H23.

H26: Enter the critical t value from the t-table in Appendix E in this cell using $df = n_1 + n_2 - 2$ to find the critical t value

H29: =(G10–G11)/H23 (no spaces between symbols)

Note that you need an open-parenthesis *before G10* and a closed-parenthesis *after G11* so that this answer of −5 is *THEN* divided by the standard error of the difference of the means of 0.97, to give a t-test value of −4.57. Use two decimal places for the t-test result (see Fig. 5.16).

DELAY IN TRANSFER COMPARISON OF TWO HEALTHCARE FACILITIES						
FACILITY A	FACILITY B					
9	8	Null hypothesis:				
21	21					
10	16	Research hypothesis:				
12	18					
15	13	Group		n	Mean	STDEV
11	20	1 FACILITY A		19	12	3
13	16	2 FACILITY B		21	17	3
9	18					
11	15					
12	17	(n-1) x STDEV1 squared				171.68
14	19					
13	20	(n2 - 1) x STDEV2 squared				188.29
10	21					
15	19	n1 + n2 – 2				38
17	18					
11	16	1/n1 + 1/n2				0.10
9	17					
10	15					
11	13	s.e.				0.97
	15					
	16					
		critical t				2.024
		t-test				-4.57
Result:						
Conclusion:						

Fig. 5.16 Two-group t-test Formula Results

Now write the following sentence in C32 to C33 to summarize the *result* of the study:

C32: Since the absolute value of −4.57 is greater than the critical t of 2.024,

C33: we reject the null hypothesis and accept the research hypothesis.

Finally, write the following sentence in C36 to C37 to summarize the *conclusion* of the study:

C36: FACILITY B took significantly more days to transfer patients to a
C37: long-term care facility than did FACILITY A (17 days vs. 12 days).

Save your file as: TRANSFER3

Print the final spreadsheet so that it fits onto one page.
Write the null hypothesis and the research hypothesis by hand on your printout.
The final spreadsheet appears in Fig. 5.17.

DELAY IN TRANSFER COMPARISON OF TWO HEALTHCARE FACILITIES

FACILITY A	FACILITY B					
9	8	Null hypothesis:		μ_1	=	μ_2
21	21					
10	16	Research hypothesis:		μ_1	≠	μ_2
12	18					
15	13	Group	n	Mean	STDEV	
11	20	1 FACILITY A	19	12	3	
13	16	2 FACILITY B	21	17	3	
9	18					
11	15					
12	17	(n-1) x STDEV1 squared			171.68	
14	19					
13	20	(n2 - 1) x STDEV2 squared			188.29	
10	21					
15	19	n1 + n2 – 2			38	
17	18					
11	16	1/n1 + 1/n2			0.10	
9	17					
10	15					
11	13	s.e.			0.97	
	15					
	16					
		critical t			2.024	
		t-test			-4.57	

Result:	Since the absolute value of – 4.57 is greater than the critical t of 2.024, we reject the null nypothesis and accept the research hypothesis.
Conclusion:	FACILITY B took significantly more days to transfer patients to a long-term care facility than did FACILITY A (17 days vs. 12 days).

Fig. 5.17 Final Spreadsheet Of Delay in Transfer Comparison of A vs. B

5.4 End-of-Chapter Practice Problems

1. The University of Missouri-St. Louis offers a Bachelor of Social Work (BSW) program that is fully-accredited by the Council on Social Work Education. This program includes 570 hours of fieldwork in a social services agency. Suppose that you have been asked to design a survey of BSW students that they will be asked to take two months before they graduate from the program. You have not decided which items to include in this survey, but you have decided to include Item #25 that asks the social work majors to rate the overall quality of the required core courses in the BSW program. Part of your analysis plan for the survey is to compare the attitudes toward the program for male majors versus female majors, and you have developed the hypothetical data below in Fig. 5.18 to test your Excel analysis skills.

BACHELOR OF SOCIAL WORK (BSW) PROGRAM

SENIOR SURVEY

Item #25: **"Overall, how would you rate the quality of the required core courses in the BSW program?**

1	2	3	4	5	6	7	8	9	10
Poor									Excellent

Males	Females
5	6
6	7
4	5
3	8
4	4
6	9
7	6
9	7
5	5
4	6
3	7
2	9
6	
5	

Fig. 5.18 Worksheet Data for Chap. 5: Practice Problem #1

(a) State the null hypothesis and the research hypothesis on an Excel spreadsheet.
(b) Find the standard error of the difference between the means using Excel
(c) Find the critical t value using Appendix E, and enter it on your spreadsheet.

(d) Perform a t-test using Excel. What is the value of t that you obtain?
Use three decimal places for all figures in the formula section of your spreadsheet.
(e) State your result on your spreadsheet.
(f) State your conclusion in plain English on your spreadsheet.
(g) Save the file as: BSW3

2. Suppose that your clinic has recently completed an alcohol treatment program in which one group consisted of males and the other group consisted of females. Part of the outcome measure of this program includes a survey of participants after the program is completed. Item #15 of this outcome survey asks participants who have completed this treatment program to rate the overall effectiveness of the alcohol treatment program on a 7-point rating scale. You want to test your Excel skills on this item and so you have created the hypothetical data given in Fig. 5.19.

ALCOHOL TREATMENT PROGRAM OUTCOME MEASURE

OVERALL PROGRAM EFFECTIVENESS RATING

Item #15: "Overall, how would you rate the effectiveness of this alcohol treatment program?

1	2	3	4	5	6	7
low						high

MALES	FEMALES
5	5
6	4
7	3
4	6
3	7
6	5
5	6
8	4
4	8
5	5
6	4
4	
5	

Fig. 5.19 Worksheet Data for Chap. 5: Practice Problem #2

(a) State the null hypothesis and the research hypothesis on an Excel spreadsheet.
(b) Find the standard error of the difference between the means using Excel
(c) Find the critical t value using Appendix E, and enter it on your spreadsheet.
(d) Perform a t-test using Excel. What is the value of t that you obtain?
(e) State your result on your spreadsheet.
(f) State your conclusion in plain English on your spreadsheet.
(g) Save the file as: ALCOHOL16

3. Suppose that the Director of a Master's program in Social Work (MSW) at Washington University in St. Louis, Missouri USA wants to determine if there is a difference in GPAs between Male students and Female students who have completed all of the required core courses in the program. Suppose, further, that the Director has obtained this data from the Registrar and has promised to keep the information confidential. You have been asked to analyze the data using your Excel skills. Assume that you have been working on this analysis, and you have determined that the 47 Males in the program have an average GPA of 3.15 with a standard deviation of 0.42, while the 56 Females in the program have an average GPA of 3.45 with a standard deviation of 0.37. You now want to analyze these data.

   (a) State the null hypothesis and research hypothesis on a separate sheet of paper.
   (b) Find the standard error of the difference between the means using ExceL
   (c) Find the critical t value using Appendix E, and enter it on your spreadsheet.
   (d) Perform a t-test using Excel. What is the value of t that you obtain?
   (e) Use 3 decimals for all figures that require a formula.
   (f) State your result on your spreadsheet.
   (g) State your conclusion in plain English on your spreadsheet.
   (h) Save the file as: MSW12

References

Bowers D. Medical statistics from scratch: an introduction for health professionals. 2nd ed. Hoboken: John Wiley & Sons; 2008.

Keller G. Statistics for management and economics. 8th ed. Mason: South-Western Cengage Learning; 2009.

Wheater C, Cook P. Using statistics to understand the environment. New York: Routledge; 2000.

Chapter 6
Correlation and Simple Linear Regression

There are many different types of "correlation coefficients," but the one we will use in this book is the Pearson product-moment correlation which we will call: *r*.

6.1 What Is a "Correlation?"

Basically, a correlation is a number between −1 and +1 that summarizes the relationship between two variables, which we will call X and Y.

A correlation can be either positive or negative. *A positive correlation means that as X increases, Y increases. A negative correlation means that as X increases, Y decreases.* In statistics books, this part of the relationship is called the *direction* of the relationship (i.e., it is either positive or negative).

The correlation also tells us the *magnitude* of the relationship between X and Y. As the correlation approaches closer to +1, we say that the relationship is *strong and positive*.

As the correlation approaches closer to −1, we say that the relationship is *strong and negative*.

A zero correlation means that there is no relationship between X and Y. This means that neither X nor Y can be used as a predictor of the other.

A good way to understand what a correlation means is to see a "picture" of the scatterplot of data points produced in a chart. Let's suppose that you want to know if variable X can be used to predict variable Y. We will place *the predictor variable X on the x-axis* (the horizontal axis of a chart) and *the dependent (criterion) variable Y on the y-axis* (the vertical axis of a chart). Suppose, further, that you have collected data given in the scatterplots below (see Fig. 6.1 through Fig. 6.6).

Figure 6.1 shows the scatterplot for a perfect positive correlation of $r = +1.0$. This means that you can perfectly predict each y-value from each x-value because the data points move "upward-and-to-the-right" along a perfectly-fitting straight line (see Fig. 6.1)

T.J. Quirk, S. Cummings, *Excel 2016 for Social Work Statistics*, Excel for Statistics,
DOI 10.1007/978-3-319-66221-3_6

X	Y
1	1
2	2
3	3
4	4
5	5
6	6

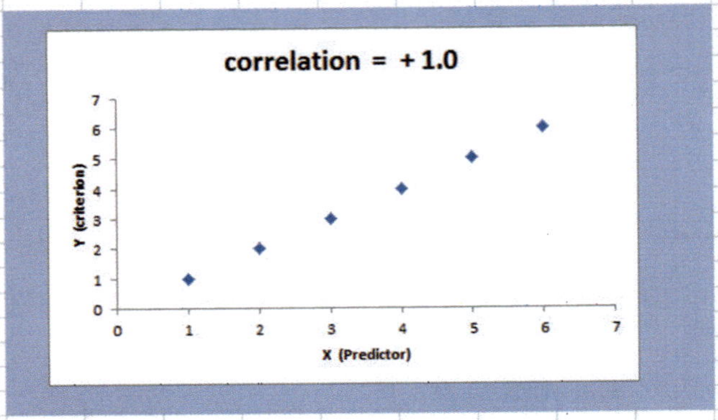

Fig. 6.1 Example of a Scatterplot for a Perfect, Positive Correlation (r = +1.0)

Figure 6.2 shows the scatterplot for a moderately positive correlation of $r = +54$. This means that each x-value can predict each y-value moderately well because you can draw a picture of a "football" around the outside of the data points that move upward-and-to-the-right, but not along a straight line (see Fig. 6.2).

X	Y
1	2
2	4
3	3
4	1
5	6
6	5

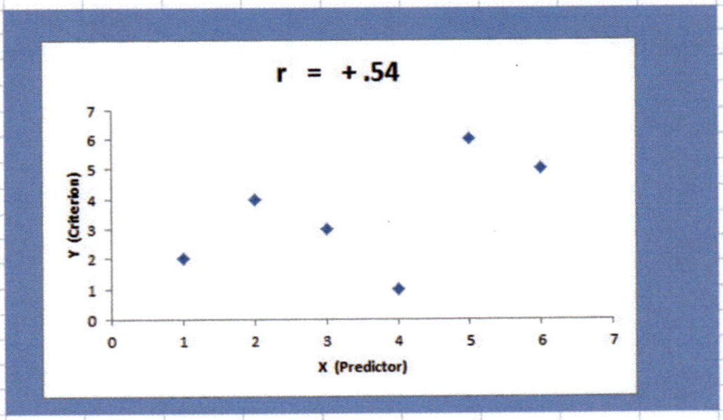

Fig. 6.2 Example of a Scatterplot for a Moderate, Positive Correlation (r = +.54)

Figure 6.3 shows the scatterplot for a low, positive correlation of $r = +.09$. This means that each x-value is a poor predictor of each y-value because the "picture" you could draw around the outside of the data points approaches a circle in shape (see Fig. 6.3)

X	Y
1	2
2	4
3	6
4	1
5	5
6	3

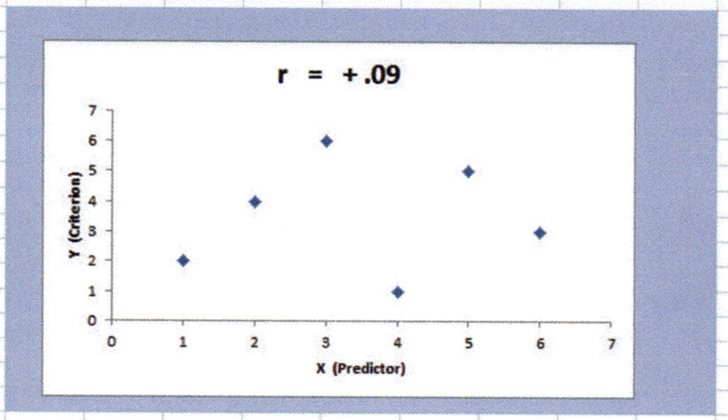

Fig. 6.3 Example of a Scatterplot for a Low, Positive Correlation (r = +.09)

We have not shown a Figure of a zero correlation because it is easy to imagine what it looks like as a scatterplot. A zero correlation of $r = .00$ means that there is no relationship between X and Y and the "picture" drawn around the data points would be a perfect circle in shape, indicating that you cannot use X to predict Y because these two variables are not correlated with one another.

Figure 6.4 shows the scatterplot for a low, negative correlation of $r = -.09$ which means that each X is a poor predictor of Y in an inverse relationship, meaning that as X increases, Y decreases (see Fig. 6.4). In this case, it is a negative correlation because the "football" you could draw around the data points slopes down and to the right.

X	Y
1	3
2	5
3	1
4	6
5	4
6	2

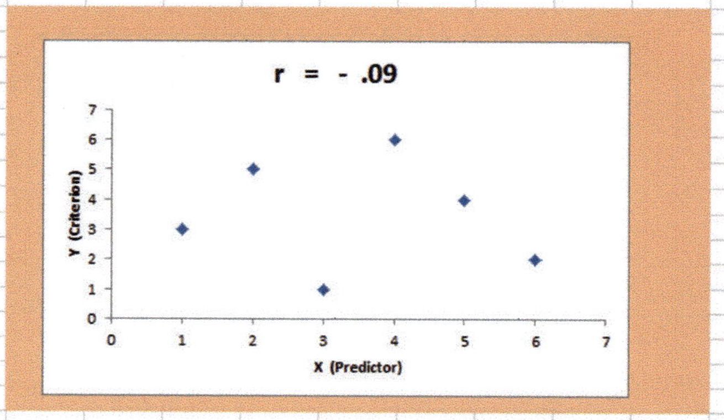

Fig. 6.4 Example of a Scatterplot for a Low, Negative Correlation (r = −.09)

Figure 6.5 shows the scatterplot for a moderate, negative correlation of $r = -.54$ which means that X is a moderately good predictor of Y, although there is an inverse relationship between X and Y (i.e., as X increases, Y decreases; see Fig. 6.5). In this case, it is a negative correlation because the "football" you could draw around the data points slopes down and to the right.

X	Y
1	5
2	6
3	1
4	3
5	4
6	2

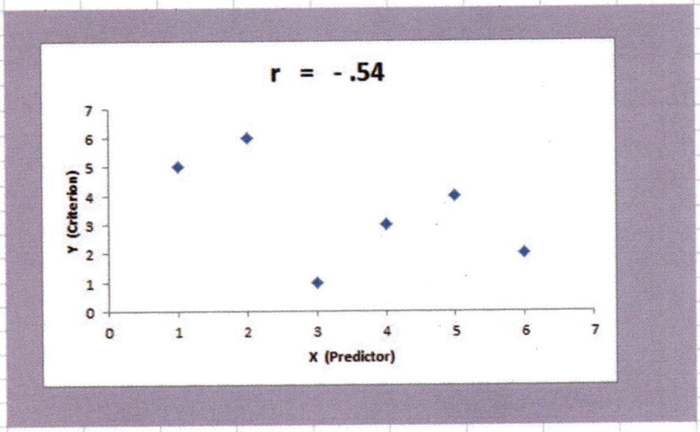

Fig. 6.5 Example of a Scatterplot for a Moderate, Negative Correlation (r = −.54)

Figure 6.6 shows a perfect negative correlation of $r = -1.0$ which means that X is a perfect predictor of Y, although in an inverse relationship such that as X increases, Y decreases. The data points fit perfectly along a downward-sloping straight line (see Fig. 6.6)

X	Y
1	6
2	5
3	4
4	3
5	2
6	1

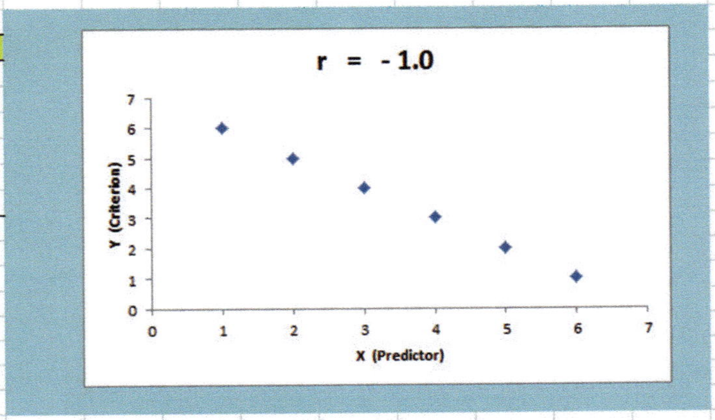

Fig. 6.6 Example of a Scatterplot for a Perfect, Negative Correlation (r = −1.0)

Let's explain the formula for computing the correlation *r* so that you can understand where the number summarizing the correlation came from.

In order to help you to understand *where* the correlation number that ranges from −1.0 to +1.0 comes from, we will walk you through the steps involved in using the formula as if you were using a calculator. This is the one time in this book that we will ask you to use your calculator to find a correlation. Knowing how a correlation is computed step-by-step will give you the opportunity to understand *how* the formula works in practice.

To do that, let's create a situation in which you need to find the correlation between two variables.

Suppose you wanted to find out if there was a relationship between high school grade-point average (HSGPA) and freshman GPA (FROSH GPA) for Social Work majors at a major university. You have decided to call HSGPA the X-variable (i.e., the predictor variable) and FROSH GPA as the Y-variable (i.e., the criterion variable) in your analysis. To test your Excel skills, you take a random sample of freshmen Social Work majors at the end of their freshman year and record their GPA. The hypothetical data for eight students appear in Fig. 6.7. *(Note: We are using only one decimal place for the GPAs in this example to simplify the mathematical computations).*

Fig. 6.7 Worksheet Data for High School GPA and Frosh GPA (Practical Example)

	A	B	C
1			
2		X	Y
3	Student	High School GPA	FROSH GPA
4	1	2.8	2.9
5	2	2.5	2.8
6	3	3.1	2.8
7	4	3.5	3.2
8	5	2.4	2.6
9	6	2.6	2.3
10	7	2.4	2.1
11	8	3.6	3.2
12			
13	n	8	8
14	MEAN	2.86	2.74
15	STDEV	0.48	0.39

Notice also that we have used Excel to find the sample size for both variables, X and Y, and the MEAN and STDEV of both variables. (You can practice your Excel skills by seeing if you get the same results when you create an Excel spreadsheet for these data.)

Now, let's use the above table to compute the correlation *r* between HSGPA and FROSH GPA using your calculator.

6.1.1 *Understanding the Formula for Computing a Correlation*

Objective: To understand the formula for computing the correlation r

The formula for computing the correlation *r* is as follows:

$$r = \frac{\frac{1}{n-1}\sum\left(X-\bar{X}\right)\left(Y-\bar{Y}\right)}{S_x\,S_y} \tag{6.1}$$

This formula looks daunting at first glance, but let's "break it down into its steps" to understand how to compute the correlation r.

6.1.2 *Understanding the Nine Steps for Computing a Correlation, r*

Objective: To understand the nine steps of computing a correlation r

The nine steps are as follows:

Step	Computation	Result
1	Find the sample size n by noting the number of students	8
2	Divide the number 1 by the sample size minus 1 (i.e., 1/7)	0.14286
3	*For each student*, take the HSGPA and subtract the meanHSGPA for the 8 students and call this $X-\bar{X}$(For example, for student # 6, this would be:2.6 − 2.86)	−0.26
	Note: With your calculator, this difference is −0.26, but whenExcel uses 16 decimal places for every computation,this result could be slightly different for each student	
4	*For each student*, take the FRGPA and subtract the meanFRGPA for the 8 students and call this $Y-\bar{Y}$(For example, for student # 6, this would be:2.3 − 2.74)	−0.44
5	Then, *for each student*, multiply $(X-\bar{X})$ times $(Y-\bar{Y})$For example, for student #6 this would be:(−0.26) × (−0.44)	+0.1144
6	Add the results of $(X-\bar{X})$ times $(Y-\bar{Y})$ for the 8 students	+1.09

Steps 1–6 would produce the Excel table given in Fig. 6.8.

	A	B	C	D	E	F	G
1							
2		X	Y				
3	Student	High School GPA	FROSH GPA	$X-\bar{X}$	$Y-\bar{Y}$	$(X-\bar{X})(Y-\bar{Y})$	
4	1	2.8	2.9	-0.06	0.16	-0.01	
5	2	2.5	2.8	-0.36	0.06	-0.02	
6	3	3.1	2.8	0.24	0.06	0.01	
7	4	3.5	3.2	0.64	0.46	0.29	
8	5	2.4	2.6	-0.46	-0.14	0.06	
9	6	2.6	2.3	-0.26	-0.44	0.11	
10	7	2.4	2.1	-0.46	-0.64	0.29	
11	8	3.6	3.2	0.74	0.46	0.34	
12						-------	
13	n	8	8		Total	1.09	
14	MEAN	2.86	2.74				
15	STDEV	0.48	0.39				

Fig. 6.8 Worksheet for Computing the Correlation, r

Notice that when Excel multiplies a negative number by a negative number, the result is a positive number (for example for student #7: (−0.46) × (−0.64) = +0.29. And when Excel multiplies a negative number by a positive number, the result is a negative number (for example for student #1: (−0.06) × (+0.16) = −0.01).

Note: Excel computes all calculations to 16 decimal places. So, when you check your work with a calculator, you may get a slightly different answer than Excel's answer.

For example, when you compute the answer for student #2:

$(X - \bar{X}) \times (Y - \bar{Y})$ for student #2, if you use two decimal places, your calculator gives:

$$(-0.36) \times (+0.06\ ) = -0.0216 \qquad (6.2)$$

As you can see from the table, Excel's answer is −0.02 which is really *more accurate* because Excel uses 16 decimal places for every number, even though only two decimal places are shown in Fig. 6.8.

You should also note that when you do Step 6, you have to be careful to add all of the positive numbers first to get *+1.10* and then add all of the negative numbers second to get *−0.03*, so that when you subtract these two numbers you get *+1.07* as your answer to Step 6. When you do these computations using Excel, this total figure will be *+1.09* because Excel carries every number and computation out to 16 decimal places which is more accurate than your calculator.

Step		
7	Multiply the answer for step 2 above by the answer for step 6(0.14286 × 1.09)	0.1557
8	Multiply the STDEV of X times the STDEV of Y(0.48 × 0.39)	0.1872
9	Finally, divide the answer from step 7 by the answer from step 8(0.1557 divided by 0.1872)	+0.83

This number of *0.83* is the correlation between HSGPA (X) and FRGPA (Y) for these 8 students. The number +*0.83* means that there is a strong, positive correlation between these two variables. That is, as HSGPA increases, FRGPA increases. For a more detailed discussion of correlation, see Weinbach and Grinnell (2010) and Rosenthal (2012).

You could also use the results presented in Fig. 6.8 in the formula for computing the correlation r in the following way:

$$\text{correlation r} = \left[(1/(\text{n}-1)) \times \sum \left(X-\bar{X}\right)\left(Y-\bar{Y}\right)\right] / \left(\text{STDEV}_\text{x} \times \text{STDEV}_\text{y}\right)$$

$$\text{correlation r} = [\,(1/7) \times 1.09]/[(.48) \times (.39)]$$

$$\text{correlation} = \text{r} = 0.83$$

When you use Excel for these computations, you obtain a slightly different correlation of +0.82 because Excel uses 16 decimal places for all numbers and computations and is, therefore, more accurate than your calculator.

Now, let's discuss how you can use Excel to find the correlation between two variables in a much simpler, and much faster, fashion than using your calculator.

6.2 Using Excel to Compute a Correlation Between Two Variables

Objective: To use Excel to find the correlation between two variables

Suppose that the financial manager of a clinic has asked you to determine the relationship between the number of visits per week to the clinic and the number of laboratory tests run that same week in the clinic.

To test your Excel skills, you have organized the resulting data into a table in which the number of visits to the clinic for each week over the past three months was recorded along with the number of lab tests run for that same week. The hypothetical data appear in Fig. 6.9.

CLINIC VISITS vs. LABTESTS

Is there a relationship between the number of visits to the clinic in a week and the number of laboratory tests run that week by the clinic?

CLINIC VISITS	LAB TESTS
60	90
64	94
68	101
72	126
64	134
79	128
82	155
85	149
76	138
66	131
69	124
85	160

Fig. 6.9 Worksheet Data for Clinic Visits and Lab Tests (Practical Example)

You want to determine if there is a *relationship* between the number of visits to the clinic each week and the number of lab tests run that same week, and you decide to use a correlation to determine this relationship. Let's call the visits to the clinic as the predictor, X, and the number of lab tests as the criterion, Y.

Create an Excel spreadsheet with the following information:

A3: CLINIC VISITS vs. LAB TESTS
B5: Is there a relationship between the number of visits to the clinic in a week and
B6: the number of laboratory tests run that week by the clinic?
B8: CLINIC VISITS
C8: LAB TESTS
B9: 60
C9: 90

Next, change the width of Columns B and C so that the information fits inside the cells.

Now, complete the remaining figures in the table given above so that B20 is 85 and C20 is 160. (Be sure to double-check your figures to make sure that they are correct!) Then, center the information in all of these cells.

A22: n
A23: mean
A24: stdev

Next, define the "name" to the range of data from B9:B20 as: VISITS

We discussed earlier in this book (see Sect. 1.4.4) how to "name a range of data," but here is a reminder of how to do that:

To give a "name" to a range of data:

Click on the top number in the range of data and drag the mouse down to the bottom number of the range.

For example, to give the name: "VISITS" to the cells: B9:B20, click on B9, and drag the pointer down to B20 so that the cells B9:B20 are highlighted on your computer screen. Then, click on:

Formulas
Define name (top center of your screen)
VISITS (enter this in the Name box; see Fig. 6.10)

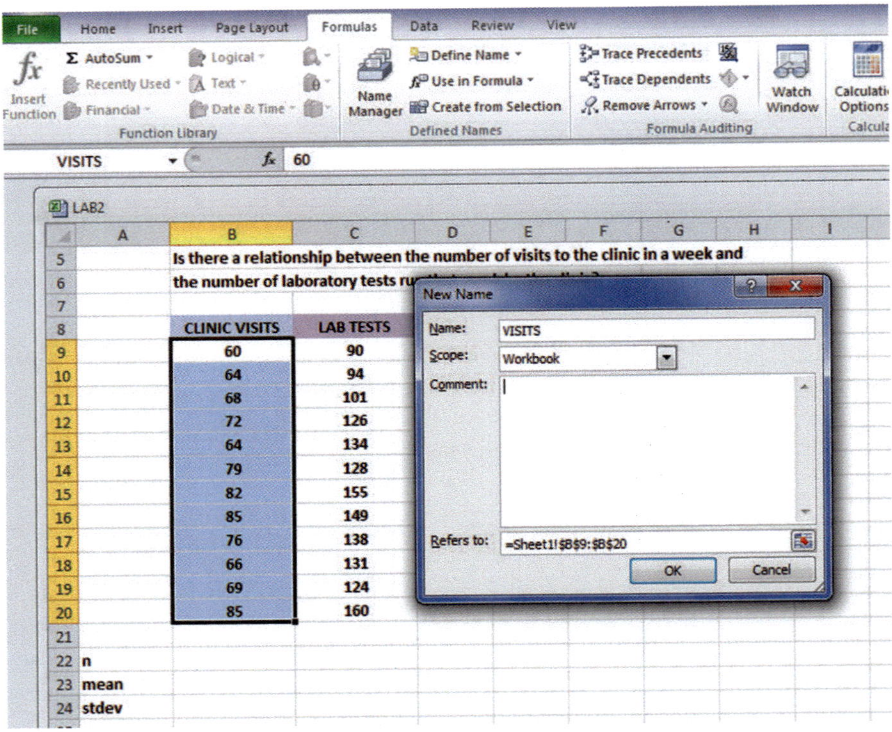

Fig. 6.10 Dialogue Box for Naming a Range of Data as: "VISITS"

OK

Now, repeat these steps to give the name: LAB to C9:C20

Finally, click on any blank cell on your spreadsheet to "deselect" cells C9:C20 on your computer screen.

Now, complete the data for these sample sizes, means, and standard deviations in columns B and C so that B23 is 72.50, and C24 is 22.73 (use two decimals for the means and standard deviations; see Fig. 6.11)

CLINIC VISITS vs. LAB TESTS

Is there a relationship between the number of visits to the clinic in a week and the number of laboratory tests run that week by the clinic?

	CLINIC VISITS	LAB TESTS
	60	90
	64	94
	68	101
	72	126
	64	134
	79	128
	82	155
	85	149
	76	138
	66	131
	69	124
	85	160
n	12	12
mean	72.50	127.50
stdev	8.70	22.73

Fig. 6.11 Example of Using Excel to Find the Sample Size, Mean, and STDEV

Objective: Find the correlation between VISITS and LAB

B26: correlation
C26: =correl(VISITS,LAB) ; see Fig. 6.12

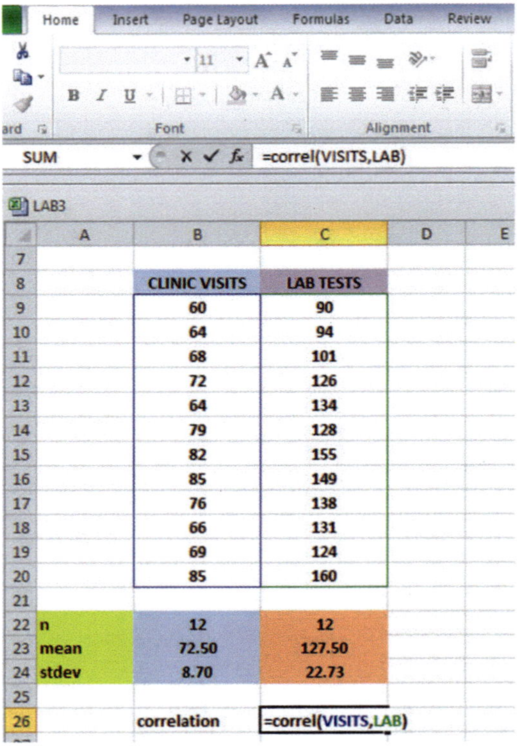

Fig. 6.12 Example of Using Excel's =correl Function to Compute the Correlation Coefficient

Hit the Enter key to compute the correlation

C26: format this cell to two decimals

Note that the equal sign in =correl(VISITS,LAB) in C26 tells Excel that you are going to use a formula in this cell.

The correlation between VISITS (X) and LAB (Y) is +*.82*, a very strong positive correlation. This means that you have evidence that there is a strong relationship between these two variables. In effect, the higher the number of visits to the clinic in a week, the more laboratory tests run that same week by the clinic.

Save this file as: LAB4

The final spreadsheet appears in Fig. 6.13.

CLINIC VISITS vs. LAB TESTS		
	Is there a relationship between the number of visits to the clinic in a week and the number of laboratory tests run that week by the clinic?	
	CLINIC VISITS	LAB TESTS
	60	90
	64	94
	68	101
	72	126
	64	134
	79	128
	82	155
	85	149
	76	138
	66	131
	69	124
	85	160
n	12	12
mean	72.50	127.50
stdev	8.70	22.73
	correlation	0.82

Fig. 6.13 Final Result of Using the =correl Function to Compute the Correlation Coefficient

6.3 Creating a Chart and Drawing the Regression Line onto the Chart

This section deals with the concept of "linear regression." Technically, the use of a simple linear regression model (i.e., the word "simple" means that only one predictor, X, is used to predict the criterion, Y) requires that the data meet the following four assumptions:

1. The underlying relationship between the two variables under study (X and Y) is *linear* in the sense that a straight line, and not a curved line, can fit the data points on the chart.
2. The errors of measurement are independent of each other (e.g. the errors from a specific time period are sometimes correlated with the errors in a previous time period).
3. The errors fit a normal distribution of Y-values at each of the X-values.
4. The variance of the errors is the same for all X-values (i.e., the variability of the Y-values is the same for both low and high values of X).

A detailed explanation of these assumptions is beyond the scope of this book, but the interested reader can find a detailed discussion of these assumptions in Levine et al. (2011, pp. 529–530).

Now, let's create a chart summarizing these data.

Important note: *Whenever you draw a chart, it is ESSENTIAL that you put the predictor variable (X) on the left, and the criterion variable (Y) on the right in your Excel spreadsheet, so that you know which variable is the predictor variable and which variable is the criterion variable. If you do this, you will save yourself a lot of grief whenever you do a problem involving correlation and simple linear regression using Excel!*

Important note: *You need to understand that in any chart that has one predictor and a criterion that there are really TWO LINES that can be drawn between the data points:(1) One line uses X as the predictor, and Y as the criterion(2) A second line uses Y as the predictor, and X as the criterion. This means that you have to be very careful to note in your input data the cells that contain X as the predictor, and Y as the criterion. If you get these cells mixed up and reverse them, you will create the wrong line for your data and you will have botched the problem terribly.This is why we STRONGLY RECOMMEND IN THIS BOOK that you always put the X data (i.e., the predictor variable) on the LEFT of your table, and the Y data (i.e., the criterion variable) on the RIGHT of your table on your spreadsheet so that you don't get these variables mixed up.*

Also note that the correlation, r, will be exactly the same correlation no matter which variable you call the predictor variable and which variable you call the criterion variable. The correlation coefficient just summarizes the relationship between two variables, and doesn't care which one is the predictor and which one is the criterion.

Let's suppose that you would like to use the number of visits to the clinic in a week as the predictor variable, and you would like to use it to predict the number of laboratory tests run that same week by the clinic. Since the correlation between these two variables is +*.82*, shows there is a strong, positive relationship and that the number of visits to the clinic in a week is a good predictor of the number of lab tests run that week by the clinic.

1. Open the file that you saved earlier in this chapter: LAB4

6.3.1 *Using Excel to Create a Chart and the Regression Line Through the Data Points*

Objective: To create a chart and the regression line summarizing the relationship between VISITS and LAB

2. Click and drag the mouse to highlight both columns of numbers (B9:C20), *but do not highlight the labels above the data points.*

Highlight the data set: B9:C20
Insert (top left of screen)
Highlight: Scatter chart icon (immediately above the word: "Charts" at the top center of your screen)
Click on the down arrow on the right of the chart icon
Highlight the top left scatter chart icon (see Fig. 6.14)

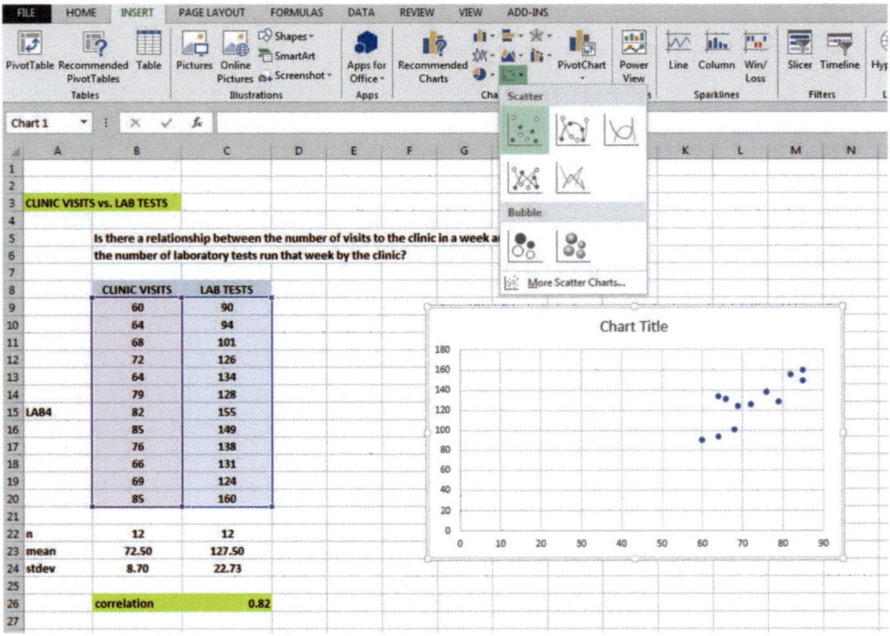

Fig. 6.14 Example of Selecting a Scatter Chart

Click on the top left chart to select it
Click on the " + icon" to the right of the chart (CHART ELEMENTS)
Click on the check mark next to "Chart Title" **and also** next to "Gridlines" to remove these check marks (see Fig. 6.15)

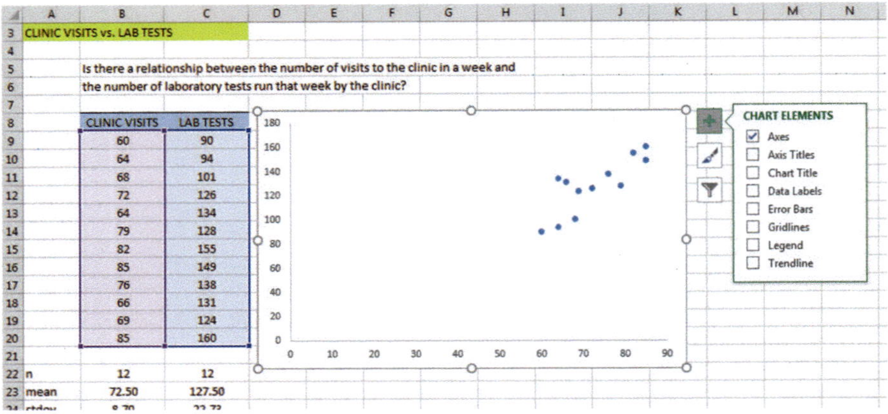

Fig. 6.15 Example of Chart Elements Selected

Click on the box next to: "Chart Title" and then click on the arrow to its right. Then, click on: "Above chart".

Note that the words: "Chart Title" are now in a box at the top of the chart (See Fig. 6.16).

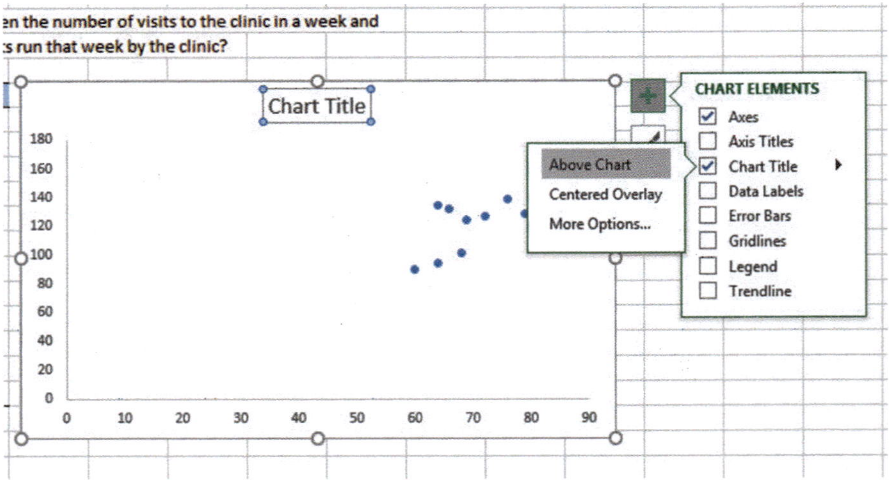

Fig. 6.16 Example of Chart Title Selected

Enter the following Chart Title to the right of $\mathbf{f_x}$ at the top of your screen: RELATIONSHIP BETWEEN CLINIC VISITS AND LAB TESTS PER WEEK (see Fig. 6.17)

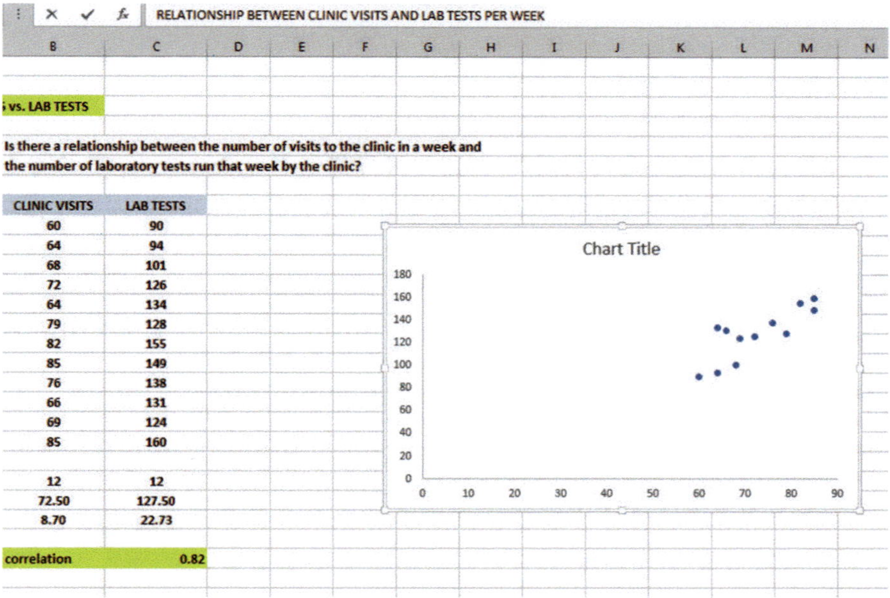

Fig. 6.17 Example of Creating a Chart Title

Hit the enter key to enter this title onto the chart

Click *inside the chart* at the top right corner of the chart to "deselect" the box around the Chart Title (see Fig. 6.18).

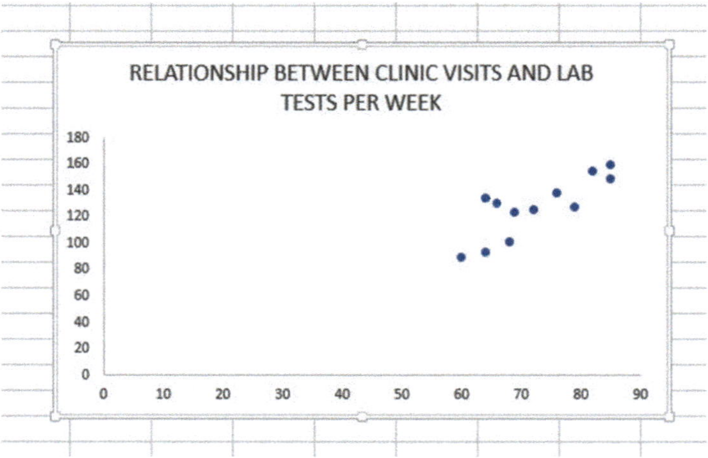

Fig. 6.18 Example of a Chart Title Inserted onto the Chart

Click on the " + box" to the right of the chart
Add a check mark to the left of "Axis Titles" (this will create an "Axis Title" box on the y-axis of the chart)
Click on the right arrow for: "Axis Titles" and then click on: "Primary Horizontal" to remove the check mark in its box (this will create the y-axis title)
Enter the following y-axis title to the right of $\mathbf{f_x}$ at the top of your screen: TESTS

Then, hit the Enter Key to enter this y-axis title onto the chart.
Click *inside the chart at the top right corner of the chart* to "deselect" the box around the y-axis title (see Fig. 6.19).

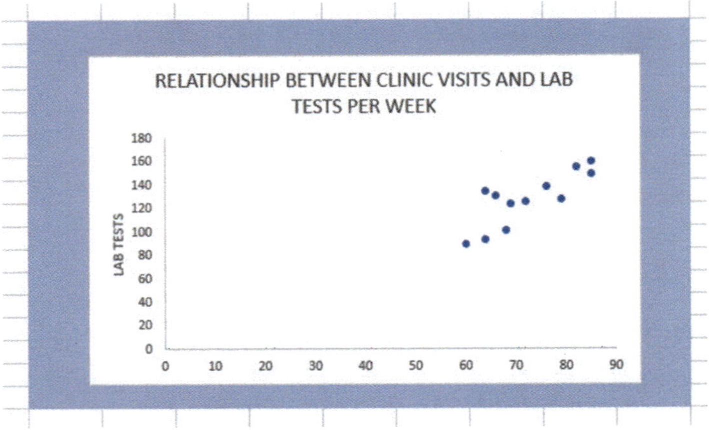

Fig. 6.19 Example of Adding a y-axis Title to the Chart

Click on the " + box" to the right of the chart
Highlight: "Axis Titles" and click on its right arrow
Click on the words: "Primary Horizontal" to add a check mark to its box (this Creates an "Axis Title" box on the x-axis of the chart)
Enter the following x-axis title to the right of $\mathbf{f_x}$ at the top of your screen: CLINIC VISITS

Then, hit the Enter Key to add this x-axis title to the chart
Click *inside the chart at the top right corner of the chart* to "deselect" the box around the x-axis title (see Fig. 6.20).

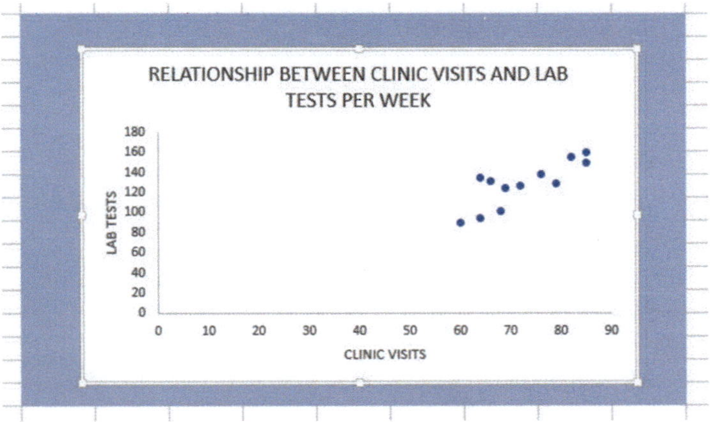

Fig. 6.20 Example of a Chart Title, an x-axis Title, and a y-axis Title

Now, let's draw the regression line onto the chart. This regression line is called the "least-squares regression line" and it is the "best-fitting" straight line through the data points.

6.3.1.1 Drawing the Regression Line Through the Data Points in the Chart

Objective: To draw the regression line through the data points on the chart

Right-click on any one of the data points inside the chart
Highlight: Add Trendline (see Fig. 6.21)

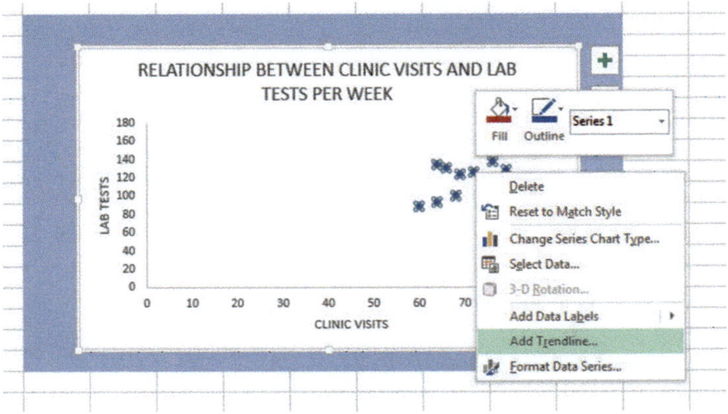

Fig. 6.21 Dialogue Box for Adding a Trendline to the Chart

Click on: Add Trendline

Linear (be sure the "linear" button near the top is selected on the "Format Trendline" dialog box; see Fig. 6.22)

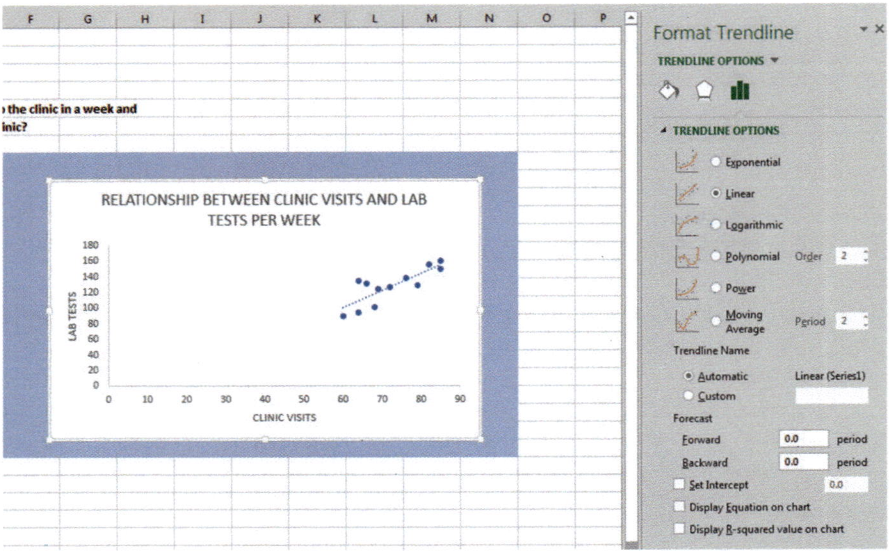

Fig. 6.22 Dialog Box for a Linear Trendline

Click on the X at the top right of the "Format Trendline" dialog box to close this dialog box

Click on any blank cell *outside the chart* to "deselect the chart"

Save this file as: LAB5

Your spreadsheet should look like the spreadsheet in Fig. 6.23.

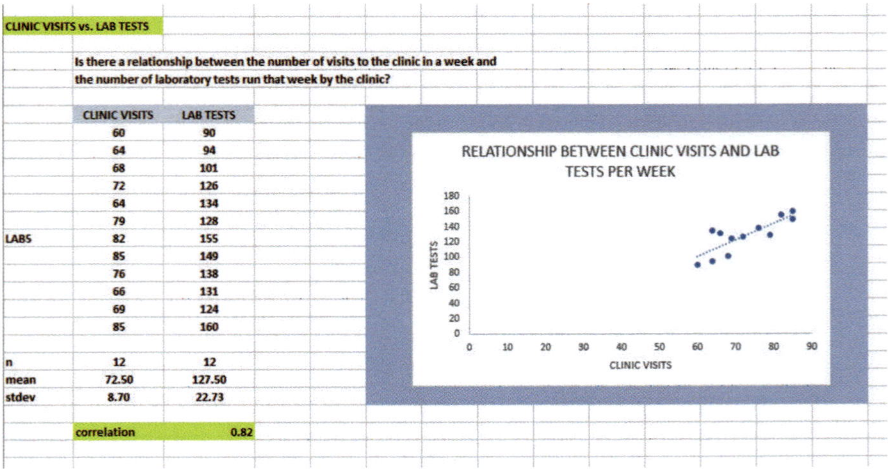

Fig. 6.23 Final Chart with the Trendline Fitted Through the Data Points of the Scatterplot

6.3.1.2 Moving the Chart Below the Table in the Spreadsheet

Objective: To move the chart below the table

Left-click your mouse on *any white space to the right of the top title inside the chart*, keep the left-click down, and drag the chart down and to the left so that the top left corner of the chart is in cell A29, then take your finger off the left-click of the mouse (see Fig. 6.24).

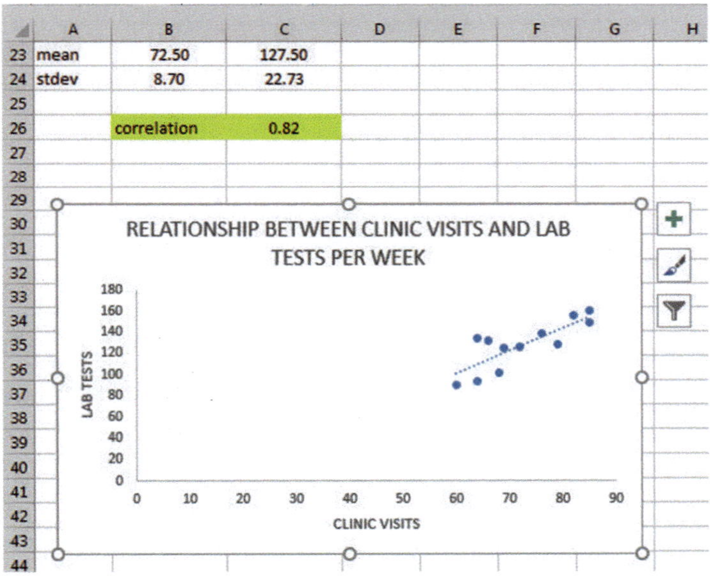

Fig. 6.24 Example of Moving the Chart Below the Table

6.3.1.3 Making the Chart "Longer" so That It Is "Taller"

Objective: To make the chart "longer" so that it is taller

Left-click your mouse on the bottom-center of the chart to create an "up-and-down-arrow" sign, hold the left-click of the mouse down and drag the bottom of the chart down to row 48 to make the chart longer, and then take your finger off the mouse.

6.3.1.4 Making the Chart "Wider"

Objective: To make the chart "wider"

Put the pointer at the middle of the right-border of the chart to create a "left-to-right arrow" sign, and then left-click your mouse and hold the left-click down while you drag the right border of the chart to the middle of Column H to make the chart wider.

Now, click on any blank cell outside the chart to "deselect" the chart (see Fig. 6.25).

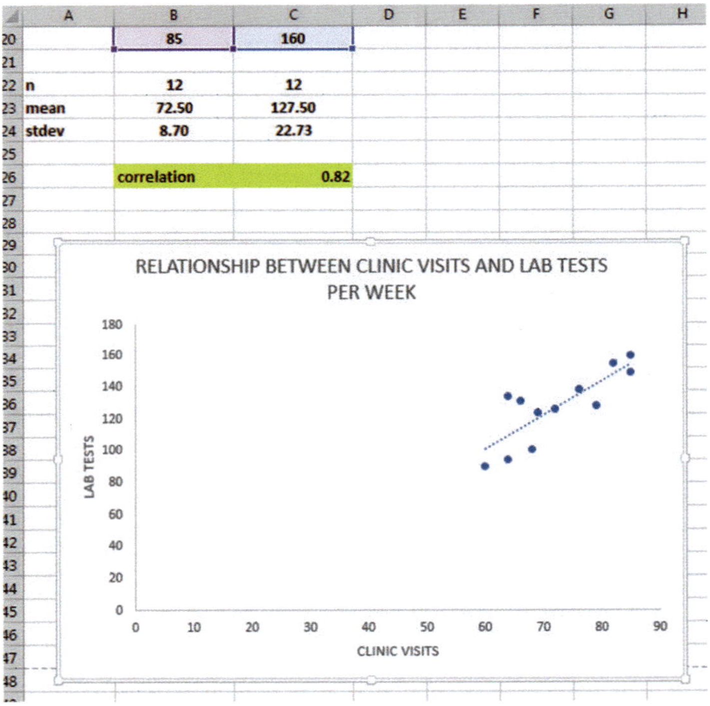

Fig. 6.25 Example of a Chart that is Enlarged to Fit the Cells: A29:H48

Save this file as: LAB6

Note: If you printed this spreadsheet now, it is "too big" to fit onto one page, and would "dribble over" onto two pages of printout because the scale needs to be reduced below 100 percent in order for this worksheet to fit onto only one page. You need to complete the steps below to print out some, or all, of this spreadsheet.

6.4 Printing a Spreadsheet So That the Table and Chart Fit onto One Page

Objective: To print the spreadsheet so that the table and the chart fit onto one page

Page Layout (top of screen)

Change the scale at the middle icon near the top of the screen "Scale to Fit" by clicking on the down-arrow until it reads "90%" so that the table and the chart will fit onto one page on your printout (see Fig. 6.26):

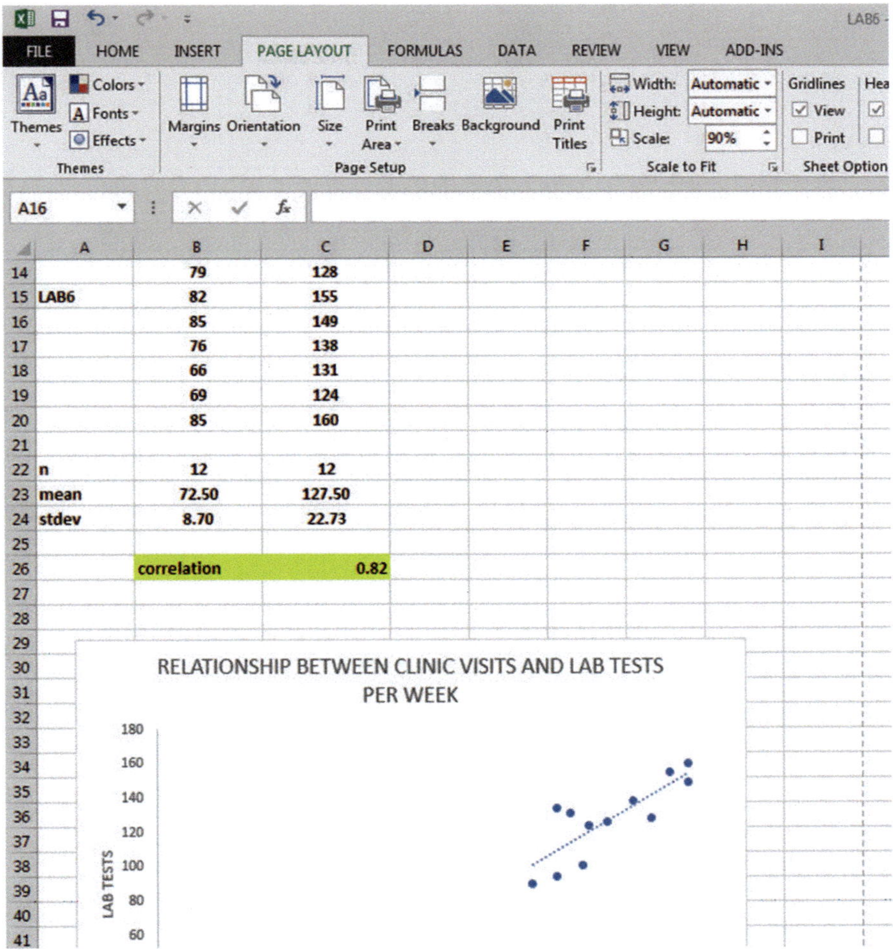

Fig. 6.26 Example of the Page Layout for Reducing the Scale of the Chart to 90% of Normal Size

File
Print
Print (see Fig. 6.27)

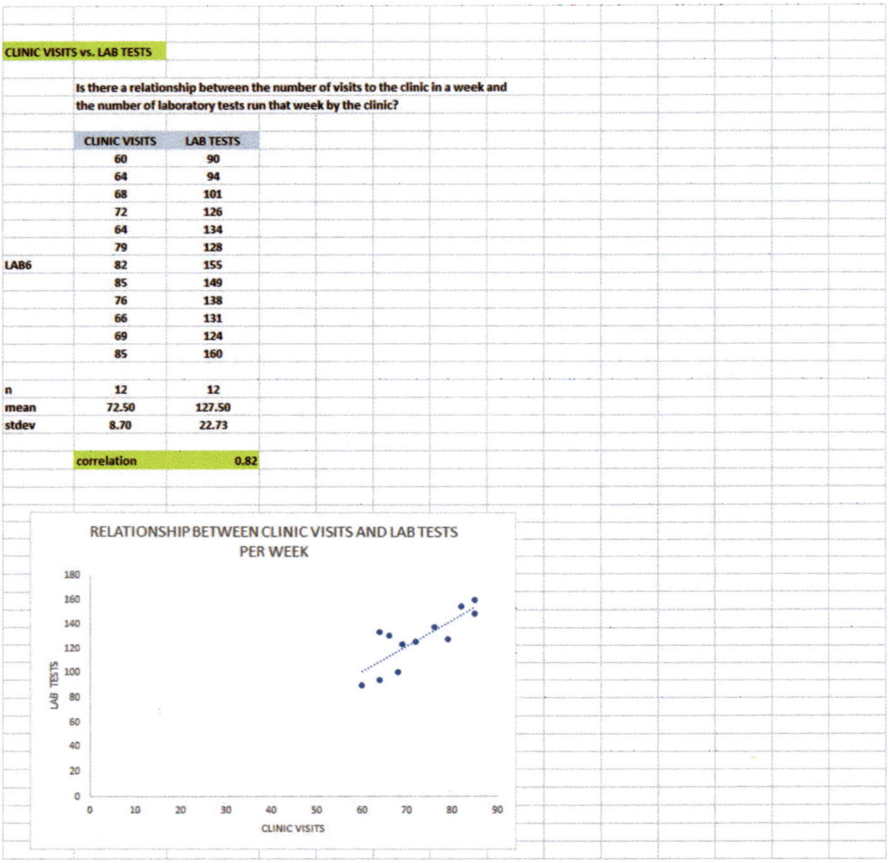

CLINIC VISITS vs. LAB TESTS

Is there a relationship between the number of visits to the clinic in a week and the number of laboratory tests run that week by the clinic?

	CLINIC VISITS	LAB TESTS
	60	90
	64	94
	68	101
	72	126
	64	134
	79	128
LAB6	82	155
	85	149
	76	138
	66	131
	69	124
	85	160
n	12	12
mean	72.50	127.50
stdev	8.70	22.73
	correlation	0.82

Fig. 6.27 Final Spreadsheet of a Table and a Chart (90% Scale to Fit Size)

Save your file as: LAB7

6.5 Finding the Regression Equation

The main reason for charting the relationship between X and Y (i.e., VISITS as X and LAB as Y in our example) is to see if there is a strong enough relationship between X and Y so that the regression equation that summarizes this relationship can be used to predict Y for a given value of X.

Since we know that the correlation between the VISITS and LAB is +*.82*, this tells us that it makes sense to use VISITS to predict LAB based on past data.

We now need to find the regression equation that is the "best-fitting straight line" through the data points.

Objective: To find the regression equation summarizing the relationship between X and Y.

In order to find this equation, we need to check to see if your version of Excel contains the "Data Analysis ToolPak" necessary to run a regression analysis.

6.5.1 Installing the Data Analysis ToolPak into Excel

Objective: To install the Data Analysis ToolPak into Excel

Since there are currently four versions of Excel in the marketplace (2007, 2010, 2013, 2016), we will give a brief explanation of how to install the Data Analysis ToolPak into each of these versions of Excel.

6.5.1.1 Installing the Data Analysis ToolPak into Excel 2016

Open a new Excel spreadsheet

Click on: Data (at the top of your screen)

Look at the top of your monitor screen. Do you see the words: "Data Analysis" at the far right of the screen? If you do, the Data Analysis ToolPak for Excel 2016 was correctly installed when you installed Office 2016, and you should skip ahead to Sect. 6.5.2.

If the words: "Data Analysis" are not at the top right of your monitor screen, then the ToolPak component of Excel 2016 was not installed when you installed Office 2016 onto your computer. If this happens, you need to follow these steps:

File
Options (bottom left of screen)
Note: This creates a dialog box with "Excel Options" at the top left of the box
Add-Ins (on left of screen)
Manage: Excel Add-Ins (at the bottom of the dialog box)
Go (at bottom center of dialog box)
Highlight: Analysis ToolPak (in the Add-Ins dialog box)
Put a check mark to the left of Analysis Toolpak

OK (at the right of this dialog box)
Data

You now should have the words: "Data Analysis" at the top right of your screen to show that this feature has been installed correctly

Note: If these steps do not work, you should try these steps instead: File/Options (bottom left)/Add-ins/Analysis ToolPak/Go/ click to the left of Analysis ToolPak to add a check mark/OK

If you need help doing this, ask your favorite "computer techie" for help.

You are now ready to skip ahead to Sect. 6.5.2

6.5.1.2 Installing the Data Analysis ToolPak into Excel 2013

Open a new Excel spreadsheet

Click on: Data (at the top of your screen)

Look at the top of your monitor screen. Do you see the words: "Data Analysis" at the far right of the screen? If you do, the Data Analysis ToolPak for Excel 2013 was correctly installed when you installed Office 2013, and you should skip ahead to Sect. 6.5.2.

If the words: "Data Analysis" are not at the top right of your monitor screen, then the ToolPak component of Excel 2013 was not installed when you installed Office 2013 onto your computer. If this happens, you need to follow these steps:

File
Options (bottom left of screen)
Note: This creates a dialog box with "Excel Options" at the top left of the box
Add-Ins (on left of screen)
Manage: Excel Add-Ins (at the bottom of the dialog box)
Go (at bottom center of dialog box)
Highlight: Analysis ToolPak (in the Add-Ins dialog box)
Put a check mark to the left of Analysis Toolpak
OK (at the right of this dialog box)
Data

You now should have the words: "Data Analysis" at the top right of your screen to show that this feature has been installed correctly

If you get a prompt asking you for the "installation CD," put this CD in the CD drive and click on: OK

Note: If these steps do not work, you should try these steps instead: File/Options (bottom left)/Add-ins/Analysis ToolPak/Go/ click to the left of Analysis ToolPak to add a check mark/OK

If you need help doing this, ask your favorite "computer techie" for help.

You are now ready to skip ahead to Sect. 6.5.2

6.5.1.3 Installing the Data Analysis ToolPak into Excel 2010

Open a new Excel spreadsheet

Click on: Data (at the top of your screen)

Look at the top of your monitor screen. Do you see the words: "Data Analysis" at the far right of the screen? If you do, the Data Analysis ToolPak for Excel 2010 was correctly installed when you installed Office 2010, and you should skip ahead to Sect. 6.5.2.

If the words: "Data Analysis" are not at the top right of your monitor screen, then the ToolPak component of Excel 2010 was not installed when you installed Office 2010 onto your computer. If this happens, you need to follow these steps:

File
Options
Excel options (creates a dialog box)
Add-Ins
Manage: Excel Add-Ins (at the bottom of the dialog box)
Go
Highlight: Analysis ToolPak (in the Add-Ins dialog box)
OK
Data (You now should have the words: "Data Analysis" at the top right of your screen)
If you get a prompt asking you for the "installation CD," put this CD in the CD drive and click on: OK

Note: *If these steps do not work, you should try these steps instead: File/Options (bottom left)/Add-ins/Analysis ToolPak/Go/ click to the left of Analysis ToolPak to add a check mark/OK*

If you need help doing this, ask your favorite "computer techie" for help.

You are now ready to skip ahead to Sect. 6.5.2.

6.5.1.4 Installing the Data Analysis ToolPak into Excel 2007

Open a new Excel spreadsheet

Click on: Data (at the top of your screen)

If the words "Data Analysis" do not appear at the top right of your screen, you need to install the Data Analysis ToolPak using the following steps:

Microsoft Office button (top left of your screen)
Excel options (bottom of dialog box)
Add-ins (far left of dialog box)
Go (to create a dialog box for Add-Ins)

Highlight: Analysis ToolPak
OK (If Excel asks you for permission to proceed, click on: Yes)
Data (You should now have the words: "Data Analysis" at the top right of your screen)

If you need help doing this, ask your favorite "computer techie" for help.
You are now ready to skip ahead to Sect. 6.5.2.

6.5.2 Using Excel to Find the SUMMARY OUTPUT of Regression

You have now installed *ToolPak*, and you are ready to find the regression equation for the "best-fitting straight line" through the data points by using the following steps:
Open the Excel file: *LAB7* (if it is not already open on your screen)

Note: If this file is already open, and there is a "border" around the chart, you need to click on any empty cell outside of the chart to deselect the chart.

Now that you have installed *Toolpak*, you are ready to find the regression equation summarizing the relationship between VISITS and LAB used in your data set.

Remember that you gave the name: *VISITS* to the X data (the predictor), and the name: *LAB* to the Y data (the criterion) in a previous section of this chapter (see Sect. 6.2)

Data (top of screen)
Data analysis (far right at top of screen; see Fig. 6.28)

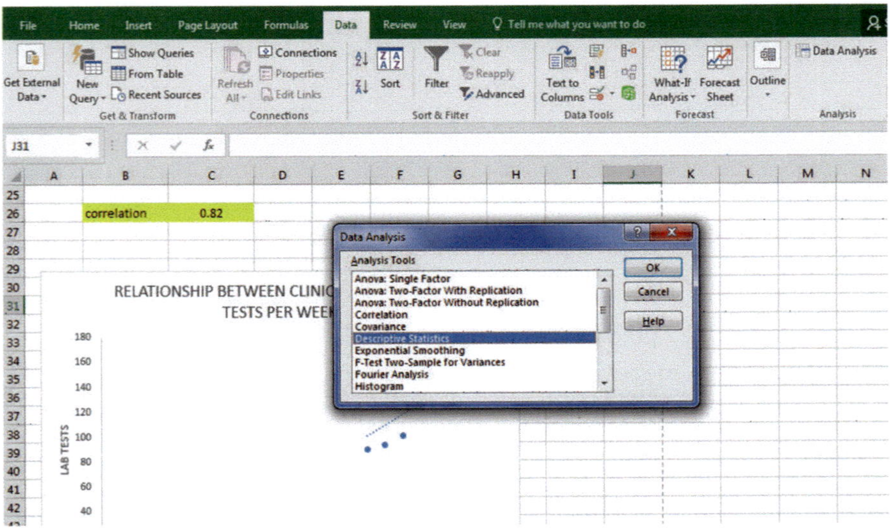

Fig. 6.28 Example of Using the Data/Data Analysis Function of Excel

Scroll down the dialog box using the down arrow and highlight: Regression (see Fig. 6.29)

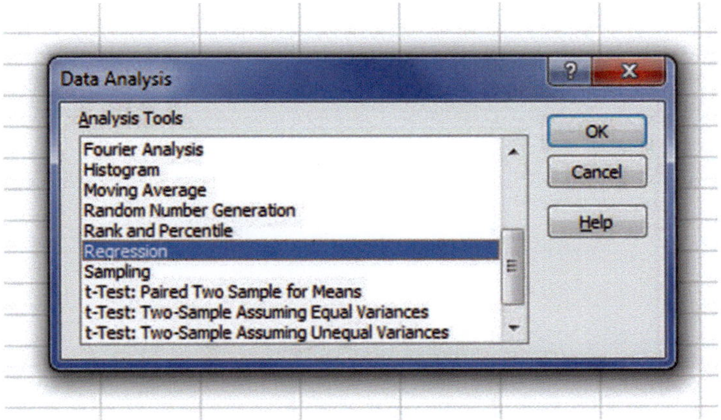

Fig. 6.29 Dialog Box for Creating the Regression Function in Excel

OK
Input Y Range: LAB
Input X Range: VISITS

Click on the "button" to the left of Output Range to select this, and enterA52 in the box as the place on your spreadsheet to insert the regression analysis in cell A52.
OK

The *SUMMARY OUTPUT* should now be in cells: A52 : I69

Now, make the columns in the Regression SUMMARY OUTPUT section of your spreadsheet *wider* so that you can read all of the column headings clearly.

Now, change the data in the following two cells to Number format (two decimal places):

B55
B68

Next, change this cell to four decimal places: B69

Now, change the format for all other numbers that are in decimal format to number format, three decimal places, and center all numbers within their cells.

Print the file so that it fits onto one page. (*Hint: Change the scale under "Page Layout" to 65% to make it fit.)* Your file should be like the file in Fig. 6.30.

CLINIC VISITS vs. LAB TESTS

Is there a relationship between the number of visits to the clinic in a week and the number of laboratory tests run that week by the clinic?

	CLINIC VISITS	LAB TESTS
	60	90
	64	94
	68	101
	72	126
	64	134
	79	128
LAB8	82	155
	85	149
	76	138
	66	131
	69	124
	85	160
n	12	12
mean	72.50	127.50
stdev	8.70	22.73
	correlation	0.82

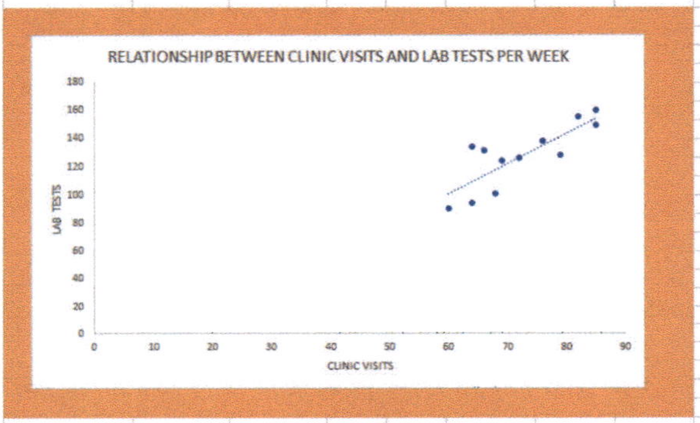

SUMMARY OUTPUT

Regression Statistics	
Multiple R	0.82
R Square	0.672
Adjusted R Square	0.639
Standard Error	13.654
Observations	12

ANOVA

	df	*SS*	*MS*	*F*	*Significance F*
Regression	1	3820.715	3820.715	20.494	0.001
Residual	10	1864.285	186.428		
Total	11	5685.000			

	Coefficients	*Standard Error*	*t Stat*	*P-value*	*Lower 95%*	*Upper 95%*	*Lower 95.0%*	*Upper 95.0%*
Intercept	-27.77	34.524	-0.804	0.440	-104.694	49.154	-104.694	49.154
X Variable 1	2.1417	0.473	4.527	0.001	1.088	3.196	1.088	3.196

Fig. 6.30 Final Spreadsheet of Correlation and Simple Linear Regression including the SUMMARY OUTPUT for the Data

Save this file as: LAB8

Note the following problem with the summary output.

Whoever wrote the computer program for this version of Excel made a mistake and gave the name: "Multiple R" to cell A55.

This is not correct. Instead, cell A55 should say: "correlation r" since this is the notation that we are using for the correlation between X and Y.

You can now use your printout of the regression analysis to find the regression equation that is the best-fitting straight line through the data points.

But first, let's review some basic terms.

6.5.2.1 Finding the y-Intercept, a, of the Regression Line

The point on the y-axis at which the regression line would intersect the y-axis if it were extended to reach the y-axis is called the "y-intercept" and *we will use the letter "a" to stand for the y-intercept of the regression line*. The y-intercept on the SUMMARY OUTPUT of Fig. 6.30 is *−27.77 (note the negative number) and appears in cell B68*. This means that if you were to draw an imaginary line continuing down the regression line toward the y-axis that this imaginary line would cross the y-axis at −27.77. This is why it is called the "y-intercept."

6.5.2.2 Finding the Slope, b, of the Regression Line

The "tilt" of the regression line is called the "slope" of the regression line. It summarizes to what degree the regression line is either above or below a horizontal line through the data points. If the correlation between X and Y were zero, the regression line would be exactly horizontal to the X-axis and would have a zero slope.

If the correlation between X and Y is positive, the regression line would "slope upward to the right" above the X-axis. Since the regression line in Fig. 6.30 slopes upward to the right, the slope of the regression line is +2.1417 as given in cell *B69*. *We will use the notation "b" to stand for the slope of the regression line*. (Note that Excel calls the slope of the line: "X Variable 1" in the Excel printout.)

Since the correlation between VISITS and LAB was +*.82*, you can see that the regression line for these data "slopes upward to the right" through the data. Note that the SUMMARY OUTPUT of the regression line in Fig. 6.30 gives a correlation, r, of +*.82* in cell *B55*.

If the correlation between X and Y were negative, the regression line would "slope down to the right" above the X-axis. This would happen whenever the correlation between X and Y is a negative correlation that is between zero and minus one (0 and −1).

6.5.3 Finding the Equation for the Regression Line

To find the regression equation for the straight line that can be used to predict the number of lab tests run in a week, we only need two numbers in the SUMMARY OUTPUT in Fig. 6.30: *B68 and B69*.

$$\text{The format for the regression line is : } \quad Y = a + b\,X \qquad (6.3)$$

where a = *the y-intercept* (−27.77 in our example in cell B68)
and b = *the slope of the line* (+2.1417 in our example in cell B69)
Therefore, the equation for the best-fitting regression line for our example is:

$$\mathrm{Y = a + b\,X}$$

$$\boxed{\mathrm{Y} = -27.77 + 2.1417\,\mathrm{X}}$$

Remember that Y is the number of lab tests run in a week that we are trying to predict, using the number of visits to the clinic that same week as the predictor, X.

Let's try an example using this formula to predict the number of lab tests run for a week.

6.5.4 Using the Regression Line to Predict the y-Value for a Given x-Value

Objective: To find the number of lab tests predicted for a week in which the clinic had 70 visits by patients

Since the number of visits is 70 that week (i.e., X = 70), substituting this number into our regression equation gives:

$$\mathrm{Y} = -27.77 + 2.1417(70)$$
$$\mathrm{Y} = -27.77 + 149.92$$
$$\mathrm{Y} = 122.15 \text{ or } 122 \text{ lab tests predicted for a week with 70 visits}$$

Important note: If you move directly upwards in your chart for CLINIC VISITS of 70 until you hit the regression line, you will see that you hit this line just ABOVE 120 on the y-axis to the left when you draw a line horizontal to the x-axis (actually, it is exactly 122.15), the result from above for predicting the number of lab tests run for a week with 70 visits to the clinic.

Now, let's do a second example and predict the number of lab tests that would result if we had 80 visits to the clinic in a week.

$$\mathrm{Y} = -27.77 + 2.1417\,\mathrm{X}$$
$$\mathrm{Y} = -27.77 + 2.1417\,(80)$$
$$\mathrm{Y} = -27.77 + 171.34$$
$$\mathrm{Y} = 143.57 \text{ or } 143 \text{ lab tests are predicted for a week with 80 visits}$$

Important note: If you move directly upwards in your chart from clinic visits of 80 until you hit the regression line, you will see that you hit this line just above 140 on the y-axis to the left (actually it is exactly 143.57), the result from above for predicting the number of lab test run in a week with 80 visits to the clinic.

For a more detailed discussion of regression, see Rosenthal (2012) and Lewis et al. (2011).

6.6 Adding the Regression Equation to the Chart

Objective: To Add the Regression Equation to the Chart

If you want to include the regression equation within the chart next to the regression line, you can do that, but a word of caution first.

Throughout this book, we are using the regression equation for one predictor and one criterion to be the following:

$$Y = a + b\,X \qquad (6.3)$$

where a = y-intercept and
b = slope of the line

See, for example, the regression equation in Sect. 6.5.3 where the y-intercept was $a = -27.77$ and the slope of the line was $b = +2.1417$ to generate the following regression equation:

$$Y = -27.77 + 2.1417\,X$$

However, Excel 2016 uses a slightly different regression equation (which is logically identical to the one used in this book) when you add a regression equation to a chart:

$$Y = b\,X + a \qquad (6.4)$$

where a = y-intercept and b = slope of the line

Note that this equation is identical to the one we are using in this book with the terms arranged in a different sequence.

For the example we used in Sect. 6.5.3, Excel 2016 would write the regression equation on the chart as:

$$Y = 2.1417\,X - 27.77$$

This is the format that will result when you add the regression equation to the chart using Excel 2016 using the following steps:

Open the file: LAB8 *(that you saved in Sect. 6.5.2)*

Click just *inside the outer border of the chart in the top right corner* to add the "border" around the chart in order to "select the chart" for changes you are about to make
Right-click on any of the data-points in the chart
Highlight: Add Trendline, and click on it to select this command
The "Linear button" near the top of the dialog box will be selected (on its left)

Scroll down this dialog box and click on: Display Equation on chart (near the bottom of the dialog box; see Fig. 6.31)

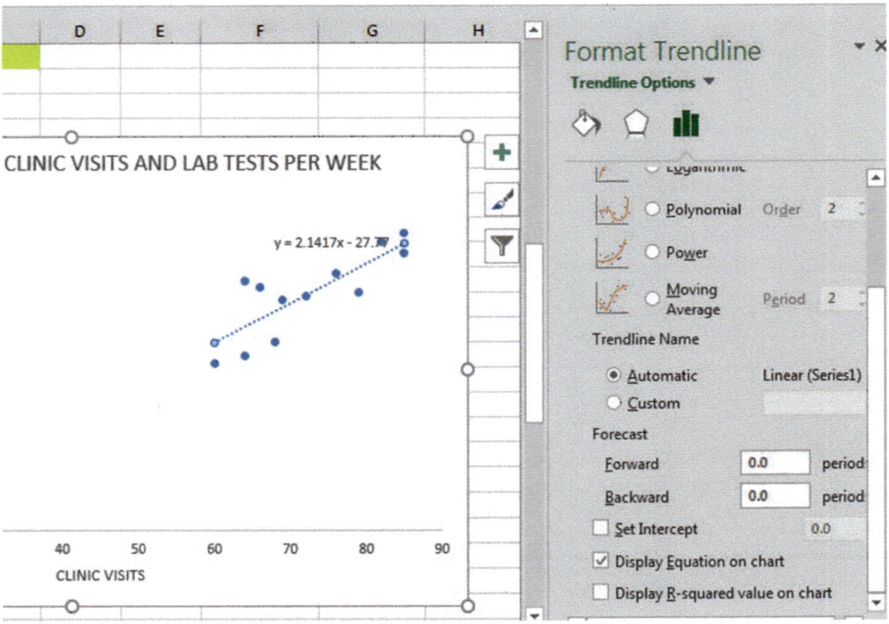

Fig. 6.31 Dialogue Box for Adding the Regression Equation to the Chart Next to the Regression Line on the Chart

Click on the X at the top right of the Format Trendline dialog box to remove this box
Click on any empty cell to deselect the chart
Note that the regression equation on the chart is in the following form next to the regression line on the chart (see Fig. 6.32).

$$Y = 2.1417\ X - 27.77$$

CLINIC VISITS vs. LAB TESTS

Is there a relationship between the number of visits to the clinic in a week and the number of laboratory tests run that week by the clinic?

	CLINIC VISITS	LAB TESTS
	60	90
	64	94
	68	101
	72	126
	64	134
	79	128
LAB8	82	155
	85	149
	76	138
	66	131
	69	124
	85	160
n	12	12
mean	72.50	127.50
stdev	8.70	22.73

correlation	0.82

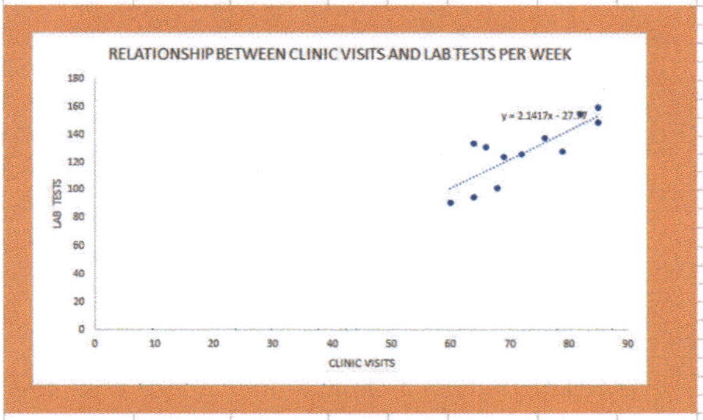

SUMMARY OUTPUT

Regression Statistics	
Multiple R	0.82
R Square	0.672
Adjusted R Square	0.639
Standard Error	13.654
Observations	12

ANOVA

	df	*SS*	*MS*	*F*	*Significance F*
Regression	1	3820.715	3820.715	20.494	0.001
Residual	10	1864.285	186.428		
Total	11	5685.000			

	Coefficients	*Standard Error*	*t Stat*	*P-value*	*Lower 95%*	*Upper 95%*	*Lower 95.0%*	*Upper 95.0%*
Intercept	-27.77	34.524	-0.804	0.440	-104.694	49.154	-104.694	49.154
X Variable 1	2.1417	0.473	4.527	0.001	1.088	3.196	1.088	3.196

Fig. 6.32 Example of a Chart with the Regression Equation Displayed Next to the Regression Line

Now, save this file as: LAB9, and print it out so that it fits onto one page

6.7 How to Recognize Negative Correlations in the SUMMARY OUTPUT Table

Important note: Since Excel does not recognize negative correlations in the SUMMARY OUTPUT results, but treats all correlations as if they were positive correlations (this was a mistake made by the programmer), you need to be careful to note that there may be a negative correlation between X and Y even if the printout says that the correlation is a positive correlation.

You will know that the correlation between X and Y is a negative correlation when these two things occur:

(1) *THE SLOPE, b, IS A NEGATIVE NUMBER. This can only occur when there is a negative correlation.*
(2) *THE CHART CLEARLY SHOWS A DOWNWARD SLOPE IN THE REGRESSION LINE, which can only occur when the correlation between X and Y is negative.*

6.8 Printing Only Part of a Spreadsheet Instead of the Entire Spreadsheet

Objective: To print part of a spreadsheet separately instead of printing the entire spreadsheet

There will be many occasions when your spreadsheet is so large in the number of cells used for your data and charts that you only want to print part of the spreadsheet separately so that the print will not be so small that you cannot read it easily.

We will now explain how to print only part of a spreadsheet onto a separate page by using three examples of how to do that using the file, LAB9, that you created in Sect. 6.6: (1) printing only the table and the chart on a separate page, (2) printing only the chart on a separate page, and (3) printing only the SUMMARY OUTPUT of the regression analysis on a separate page.

Note: If the file: LAB9 is not open on your screen, you need to open it now.

If the "border" is around the outside of the chart, click on any white space *outside of the chart* to deselect the chart.

Let's describe how to do these three goals with three separate objectives:

6.8.1 Printing Only the Table and the Chart on a Separate Page

Objective: To print only the table and the chart on a separate page

1. Left-click your mouse starting at the top left of the table *in cell A3* and drag the mouse *down and to the right so that all of the table and all of the chart are highlighted in light blue on your computer screen from cell A3 to cell H48* (the light blue cells are called the "selection" cells).
2. File
   Print
   Print Active Sheets (hit the down arrow on the right)
   Print selection
   Print

The resulting printout should contain only the table of the data and the chart resulting from the data.

Then, click on any empty cell in your spreadsheet to deselect the table and chart.

6.8.2 Printing Only the Chart on a Separate Page

Objective: To print only the chart on a separate page

1. Click on any "white space" *just inside the outside border of the chart in the top right corner of the chart* to create the "border" around all of the borders of the chart in order to "select" the chart.
2. File
   Print
   Print selected chart
   Print selected chart (again)
   Print

The resulting printout should contain only the chart resulting from the data.

Important note: Each time you print a chart by itself on a separate page, you should immediately click on any white space OUTSIDE the chart to remove the border from the chart. When the border is on the borders of the chart, this tells Excel that you want to print only the chart by itself. Do this now!

6.8.3 *Printing Only the SUMMARY OUTPUT of the Regression Analysis on a Separate Page*

Objective: To print only the SUMMARY OUTPUT of the regression analysis on a separate page

1. Left-click your mouse at the cell just above SUMMARY OUTPUT in *cell A52* on the left of your spreadsheet and drag the mouse *down and to the right* until all of the regression output is highlighted in dark blue on your screen from A52 to I69.
2. File
   Print
   Print active sheets (hit the down arrow on the right)
   Print selection
   Print

The resulting printout should contain only the SUMMARY OUTPUT of the regression analysis on a separate page.

Finally, click on any empty cell on the spreadsheet to "deselect" the regression table.

6.9 End-of-Chapter Practice Problems

1. The attitude of residents in a nursing home is an important field of study in social work service. Suppose you wanted to study the relationship between the number of extended family visits to a resident in a month and that resident's depression score on a standardized instrument at the end of that month. Is there an important relationship between these two variables? Suppose that you decided to use the CES-D Scale for a depression measure. This scale was developed by the Center for Epidemiologic studies at the National Institute of Mental Health and has been used in needs assessment studies as a self-report instrument (Royse 2010). The scale is in the public domain and can be used without permission. Each resident is asked to rate how they felt in the last week. The scale consists of 20 items (e.g. "My sleep was restless"; "I felt lonely") which are scored on the following 4-point scale:

   - Rarely or None of the Time (Less Than 1 day) is scored as: 0
   - Some or a Little of the Time (1–2 days) is scored as: 1
   - Occasionally or Moderate Amount of the Time (3–4 days) is scored as: 2
   - Most or All of the Time (5–7 days) is scored as: 3

   Total scores can range from zero to 60 such that the higher the score, the higher the depression level. Suppose that your nursing facility keeps records of extended family visits, and that you have created the hypothetical data given in Fig. 6.33.

EXTENDED FAMILY VISITS vs. DEPRESSION SCORE OF A NURSING HOME RESIDENT	
Is there a relationship between the number of visits to the nursing home by extended family members in a month and the depression score of the nursing home resident at the end of that month?	
FAMILY VISITS	DEPRESSION SCORE
0	18
2	42
4	52
3	45
5	35
7	41
6	40
8	23
9	15
10	10

Fig. 6.33 Worksheet Data for Chap. 6: Practice Problem #1

(a) create an Excel spreadsheet and chart using DEPRESSION SCORE as the criterion (dependent variable) and NO. OF EXTENDED FAMILY VISITS LAST MONTH as the predictor using the following format:

- Top title: RELATIONSHIP BETWEEN FAMILY VISITS AND DEPRESSION SCORE
- x-axis title: NO. OF EXTENDED FAMILY VISITS LAST MONTH
- y-axis title: DEPRESSION SCORE
- Re-size the chart so that it is 7 columns wide and 25 rows long
- Delete the legend
- Delete the gridlines
- Move the chart below the table

Important note: Below the table, add the word: correlation, and in the cell to its right, use the =correl function to find the correlation between these two variables. Use two decimal points for this correlation.

(b) Create the *least-squares regression line* for these data on the scatterplot. Add the regression equation to the regression line on the chart.
(c) Use Excel's *regression* function to find the equation for the least-squares regression line for these data and display the results below the chart on your spreadsheet.
(d) Use number format (two decimal places) for the correlation and also the coefficients on the SUMMARY OUTPUT, and use number format (three decimal places) for all of the other decimal figures in the SUMMARY OUTPUT.
(e) Print the input data and the chart so that this information fits onto one page.
(f) Then, print the regression output table so that this information fits onto a separate page.

(g) Save the file as: FAMILY3

Answer the following questions using your Excel printout:

1. What is the correlation r?
2. What is the y-intercept *a*?
3. What is the slope b?
4. What is the regression equation (use two decimal places for the y-intercept and the slope)?
5. Use the regression equation to predict the DEPRESSION SCORE you would expect for 5 (five) extended family visits last month.

Important note: Since Excel does not recognize negative correlations in the SUMMARY OUTPUT but treats all correlations as if they were positive correlations, you need to be careful to note when there is a negative correlation between the two variables under study.You know that the correlation is negative when:(1) The slope, b, is a negative number, which can only occur when there is a negative correlation.(2) The chart clearly shows a downward slope in the regression line, which can only happen when the correlation is negative.

2. The Director of a child protection agency is concerned with the impact of budget cuts last year which increased the caseload of child protection social workers. For the first six months of last year, the average caseload was about 35 clients per social worker. Starting in July 1 of last year, a forced budget cut increased the average caseload to about 50 clients per social worker. The Director is wondering about the relationship between caseload size and the number of sick days taken by social workers in the agency, and has asked you to collect data from employee records to determine: (1) The number of sick days in the past six months of last year for each of the 18 social workers who worked all 12 months of last year and (2) The average caseload of these social workers for the last six months of last year. You have decided to test your Excel skills, and you have created the hypothetical data given in Fig. 6.34

CASELOAD SIZE vs. NO. OF SICK DAYS IN JULY-DECEMBER OF LAST YEAR

Is there a relationship between the caseload size of workers and the number of sick days they took in the last six months of last year?

CASELOAD	NO. OF SICK DAYS
52	8
55	8
43	8
44	6
49	6
52	5
46	7
46	6
47	7
51	4
54	9
55	10
48	7
49	6
48	7
51	9
56	8
53	11

Fig. 6.34 Worksheet Data for Chap. 6: Practice Problem #2

Create an Excel spreadsheet and enter the data using CASELOAD SIZE as the independent variable (predictor) and NO. OF SICK DAYS as the dependent variable (criterion).

(a) create an *XY scatterplot* of these two sets of data such that:

- top title: RELATIONSHIP BETWEEN CASELOAD SIZE AND NO. OF SICK DAYS
- x-axis title: CASELOAD SIZE
- y-axis title: NO. OF SICK DAYS
- re-size the chart so that it is 7 columns wide and 25 rows long
- delete the legend
- delete the gridlines
- move the chart below the table

(b) Create the *least-squares regression line* for these data on the scatterplot.
(c) Use Excel to run the regression statistics to find the *equation for the least-squares regression line* for these data and display the results below the chart on your spreadsheet. Use number format (two decimal places) for the correlation, r, and also for both the y-intercept and the slope of the line. Change all other decimal figures to four decimal places.
(d) Print the input data and the chart so that this information fits onto one page.

(e) Then, print out the regression output table so that this information fits onto a separate page.

By hand:

(1a) Circle and label the value of the *y-intercept* and the *slope* of the regression line on the regression output table that you just printed.

(2b) *Estimate from the graph* the NO. OF SICK DAYS you would predict for a *CASELOAD SIZE of 50* for the last six months of last year, and write your answer in the space immediately below:

____

(f) save the file as: CASE3

Answer the following questions using your Excel printout:

1. What is the correlation?
2. What is the y-intercept?
3. What is the slope of the line?
4. What is the regression equation for these data (use two decimal places for the y-intercept and the slope)?
5. Use that regression equation to predict the NO. OF SICK DAYS you would expect for a CASELOAD of 50.

(Note that this correlation is not the multiple correlation as the Excel table indicates, but is merely the correlation r instead.)

You should have found a positive correlation of +.42 between CASELOAD SIZE and NO. OF SICK DAYS. You know that the correlation is a positive correlation for two reasons: (1) the regression line slopes upward and to the right on the chart, signaling a positive correlation, and (2) the slope is +0.19 which also tells you that the correlation is a positive correlation.

3. Suppose that you wanted to study the relationship between DIET (measured in calories allowed per day) and WEIGHT LOSS (measured in kilograms, kg) for adult women between the ages of 30 and 40 who are overweight for their height and body structure, and who all weigh roughly the same number of kilograms before undertaking the weight loss program. You want to test your Excel skills on a random sample of these women based on their weight change over the past four months to make sure that you can do this type of research. The hypothetical data appear in Fig. 6.35:

Fig. 6.35 Worksheet Data for Chap. 6: Practice Problem #3

RELATIONSHIP BETWEEN DIET AND WEIGHT LOSS	
ADULT WOMEN AGES 30-40	
DIET (calories allowed per day)	**WEIGHT LOSS (kg)**
900	16.0
1050	12.0
1150	8.0
1275	6.0
1420	3.0
1530	5.5
1610	9.5
1710	2.5
1820	6.0
1875	9.0
1930	6.0
2100	3.0

Create an Excel spreadsheet and enter the data using DIET (calories allowed per day) as the independent variable (predictor) and WEIGHT LOSS (kg) as the dependent variable (criterion). Underneath the table, use Excel's =*correl* function to find the correlation between these two variables. Label the correlation and place it underneath the table; then round off the correlation to two decimal places.

(a) create an *XY scatterplot* of these two sets of data such that:

- top title: RELATIONSHIP BETWEEN DIET AND WEIGHT LOSS
- x-axis title: DIET (calories allowed per day)
- y-axis title: WEIGHT LOSS (kg)
- move the chart below the table and the correlation
- re-size the chart so that it is 8 columns wide and 25 rows long
- delete the legend
- delete the gridlines

(b) Create the *least-squares regression line* for these data on the scatterplot, and add the regression equation to the chart.

(c) Use Excel to run the regression statistics to find the *equation for the least-squares regression line* for these data and display the results below the chart on your spreadsheet. Use number format (two decimal places) for the correlation and three decimal places for all other decimal figures, including the coefficients.

(d) Print just the input data and the chart so that this information fits onto one page. Then, print the regression output table on a separate page so that it fits onto that separate page.

(e) save the file as: DIET3

Answer the following questions using your Excel printout:

1. What is the correlation between DIET and WEIGHT LOSS?
2. What is the y-intercept?
3. What is the slope of the line?
4. What is the regression equation?
5. Use the regression equation to predict the WEIGHT LOSS you would expect for a woman who was practicing a DIET of 1500 calories allowed a day. Show your work on a separate sheet of paper.

References

Levine D, Stephan D, Krehbiel T, Berenson M. Statistics for managers using microsoft excel. 6th ed. Boston: Prentice Hall Pearson; 2011.

Lewis J B, McGrath RJ, Seidel LF. Essentials of applied quantitative methods for health services managers. Sudbury: Jones and Bartlett; 2011.

Rosenthal J. Statistics and data interpretation for social work. New York: Springer Publishing Company; 2012.

Royse D. Research methods in social work. 6th ed. Belmont CA: Cengage Learning; 2010.

Weinbach R, Grinnell Jr. R. Statistics for social workers. 8th ed. Boston: Allyn & Bacon; 2010.

Chapter 7
Multiple Correlation and Multiple Regression

There are many times in social work research when you may be able to develop a better prediction model for a dependent (criterion) variable, Y, by using *several predictors* in combination (e.g. X_1, X_2, X_3, etc.) instead of a single predictor, X.

The resulting statistical procedure is called "multiple regression" because it uses two or more predictors in combination to predict Y, instead of a single predictor, X. Each predictor is "weighted" differently based on its separate correlation with Y and its correlation with the other predictors. The job of multiple correlation is to produce a regression equation that will weight each predictor differently and in such a way that the combination of predictors does a better job of predicting Y than any single predictor by itself. We will call the multiple correlation: R_{xy}.

You will recall (see Sect. 6.5.3) that the regression equation that predicts Y when only one predictor, X, is used is:

$$Y = a + bX \tag{7.1}$$

You will remember from Chap. 6 that the correlation, r, ranges from -1 to $+1$. However, the multiple correlation, R_{xy}, only ranges from zero to plus one (0 to +1). The multiple correlation is never a negative number!

7.1 Multiple Regression Equation

The multiple regression equation follows a similar format and is:

$$Y = a + b_1X_1 + b_2X_2 + b_3X_3 + \ etc. depending\ on\ the number\ of\ predictors\ used \tag{7.2}$$

The "weight" given to each predictor in the equation is represented by the letter "b" with a subscript to correspond to the same subscript on the predictors.

T.J. Quirk, S. Cummings, *Excel 2016 for Social Work Statistics*, Excel for Statistics,
DOI 10.1007/978-3-319-66221-3_7

Important note: In order to do multiple regression, you need to have installed the "Data Analysis ToolPak" that was described in Chap. 6 (see Sect. 6.5.1). If you did not install this, you need to do so now!

Let's try a practice problem.

The Graduate Record Examination (GRE) is a standardized test that is an admissions requirement for many U.S. graduate schools that offer a Master's degree in Social Work (MSW) or a Master's degree in Health Administration (MHA). The GRE is intended to measure general academic preparedness, regardless of specialization field. The GRE test produces three subtest scores: (1) GRE VERBAL REASONING (scale 130-170), (2) GRE QUANTITATIVE REASONING (scale 130-170), and (3) ANALYTICAL WRITING (scale 0–6).

Suppose that the Director of the MHA program at a major university has heard about your new Excel skills that you are developing using this book in your Social Work Statistics course, and that this Director has asked you to "think outside the box" and to help her study the relationship between GRE VERBAL, GRE QUANTITATIVE, and GRE WRITING scores to predict the first-year GPA (FIRST-YEAR GPA) of students in the Master's of Health Administration program (MHA) at her university using last year's entering class of students in that program.

You have decided to use the three subtest scores as the predictors, X_1, X_2, and X_3 and the first-year grade-point average (FIRST-YEAR GPA) as the criterion, Y. To test your Excel skills, you have randomly selected a small group of students from last year's entering MHA class, and have recorded their scores on these variables.

Let's use the following notation:

Y	FIRST-YEAR GPA
X_1	GRE VERBAL
X_2	GRE QUANTITATIVE
X_3	GRE WRITING

Suppose, further, that you have collected the following hypothetical data summarizing these scores (see Fig. 7.1):

GRADUATE RECORD EXAMINATION (GRE)			
How well does the GRE predict first-year GPA in an MHA program?			
FIRST-YEAR GPA	GRE VERBAL	GRE QUANTITATIVE	GRE WRITING
3.25	160	161	5
3.42	156	158	4
2.85	156	157	2
2.65	154	153	1
3.65	166	166	6
3.16	159	160	3
3.56	166	163	4
2.35	155	154	2
2.86	153	154	3
2.95	158	157	4
3.15	158	159	4
3.45	160	160	5

Fig. 7.1 Worksheet Data for GRE versus FIRST-YEAR GPA (Practical Example)

Create an Excel spreadsheet for these data using the following cell reference:

A2: GRADUATE RECORD EXAMINATION (GRE)
A4: How well does the GRE predict first-year GPA in an MHA program?
A6: FIRST-YEAR GPA
A7: 3.25
B6: GRE VERBAL
C6: GRE QUANTITATIVE
D6: GRE WRITING
D18: 5

Next, change the column width to match the above table, and change all GPA figures to number format (two decimal places).

Now, fill in the additional data in the spreadsheet such that:

A18: 3.45
B18: 160
D18: 5

Then, center all numbers in your table

Important note: Be sure to double-check all of your numbers in your table to be sure that they are correct, or your spreadsheets will be incorrect.

Save this file as: GRE3

Before we do the multiple regression analysis, we need to try to make one important point very clear:

Important: *When we used one predictor, X, to predict one criterion, Y, we said that you need to make sure that the X variable is ON THE LEFT in your table, and the Y variable is ON THE RIGHT in your table so that you don't get these variables mixed up (see Sect. 6.3).*

However, in multiple regression, you need to follow this rule which is exactly the opposite:
When you use several predictors in multiple regression, it is essential that the criterion you are trying to predict, Y, be ON THE FAR LEFT, and that all of the predictors be TO THE RIGHT of the criterion, Y, in your table so that you know which variable is the criterion, Y, and which variables are the predictors. If you make this a habit, you will save yourself a lot of grief.

Notice in the table above, that the criterion Y (FIRST-YEAR GPA) is on the far left of the table, and the three predictors (GRE VERBAL, GRE QUANTITATIVE, and GRE WRITING) are to the right of the criterion variable. If you follow this rule, you will be less likely to make a mistake when conducting multiple regression.

7.2 Finding the Multiple Correlation and the Multiple Regression Equation

Objective: To find the multiple correlation and multiple regression equation using Excel.

You do this by the following commands:

Data
Click on: Data Analysis (far right top of screen)
Regression (scroll down to this in the box; see Fig. 7.2)

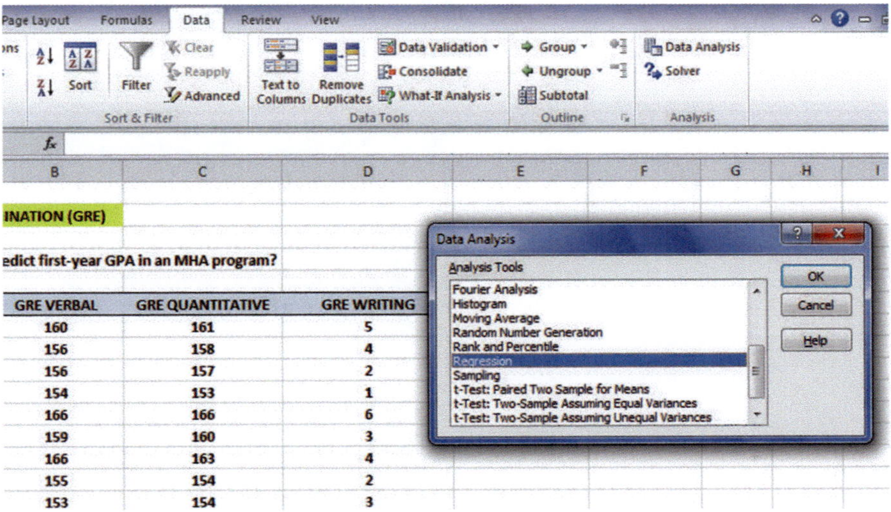

Fig. 7.2 Dialogue Box for Regression Function

OK

Input Y Range: A6:A18
Input X Range: B6:D18

Note that both the input Y Range and the Input X Range above both include the label at the top of the columns.

Click on the Labels box to *add a check mark* to it (because you have included the column labels in row 6)

Output Range (click on the button to its left, and enter): A20 (see Fig. 7.3)

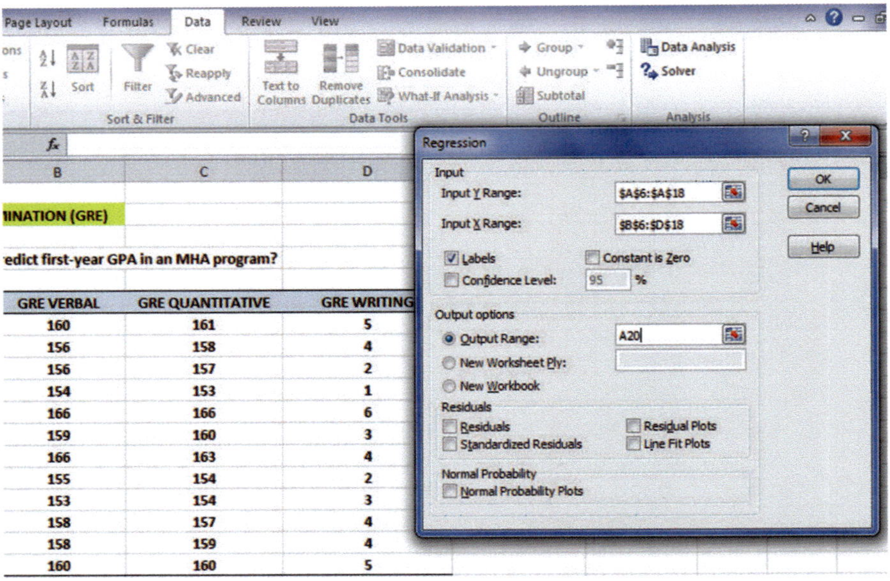

Fig. 7.3 Dialogue Box for GRE vs. FIRST-YEAR GPA Data

Important note: Excel automatically assigns a dollar sign $ in front of each column letter and each row number so that you can keep these ranges of data constant for the regression analysis.

OK (see Fig. 7.4 to see the resulting SUMMARY OUTPUT)

GRADUATE RECORD EXAMINATION (GRE)

How well does the GRE predict first-year GPA in an MHA program?

FIRST-YEAR GPA	GRE VERBAL	GRE QUANTITATIVE	GRE WRITING
3.25	160	161	5
3.42	156	158	4
2.85	156	157	2
2.65	154	153	1
3.65	166	166	6
3.16	159	160	3
3.56	166	163	4
2.35	155	154	2
2.86	153	154	3
2.95	158	157	4
3.15	158	159	4
3.45	160	160	5

SUMMARY OUTPUT

Regression Statistics	
Multiple R	0.905532671
R Square	0.819989418
Adjusted R Square	0.752485449
Standard Error	0.194101687
Observations	12

ANOVA

	df	SS	MS	F	Significance F
Regression	3	1.372962948	0.457654316	12.14727723	0.002390367
Residual	8	0.301403719	0.037675465		
Total	11	1.674366667			

	Coefficients	Standard Error	t Stat	P-value	Lower 95%
Intercept	-7.620664262	4.260893504	-1.788513197	0.111492356	-17.4463023
GRE VERBAL	-0.022937928	0.044772044	-0.512327035	0.622263259	-0.126182446
GRE QUANTITATIVE	0.088853291	0.059724909	1.487709111	0.175144874	-0.048872596
GRE WRITING	0.078000329	0.075711817	1.030226623	0.333041348	-0.096591433

Fig. 7.4 Regression SUMMARY OUTPUT of GRE vs. FIRST-YEAR GPA Data

Next, format cell B23 in number format (two decimal places)

Next, format the following four cells in Number format (three decimal places):

B36

B37

B38

B39

Change all other decimal figures to four decimal places, and center all figures within their cells.

Re-save the file as: GRE3

Now, print the file so that it fits onto one page by changing the scale to *60% size*. The resulting regression analysis is given in Fig. 7.5.

GRADUATE RECORD EXAMINATION (GRE)

How well does the GRE predict first-year GPA in an MHA program?

FIRST-YEAR GPA	GRE VERBAL	GRE QUANTITATIVE	GRE WRITING
3.25	160	161	5
3.42	156	158	4
2.85	156	157	2
2.65	154	153	1
3.65	166	166	6
3.16	159	160	3
3.56	166	163	4
2.35	155	154	2
2.86	153	154	3
2.95	158	157	4
3.15	158	159	4
3.45	160	160	5

SUMMARY OUTPUT

Regression Statistics	
Multiple R	0.91
R Square	0.8200
Adjusted R Square	0.7525
Standard Error	0.1941
Observations	12

ANOVA

	df	*SS*	*MS*	*F*	*Significance F*
Regression	3	1.3730	0.4577	12.1473	0.0024
Residual	8	0.3014	0.0377		
Total	11	1.6744			

	Coefficients	*Standard Error*	*t Stat*	*P-value*	*Lower 95%*
Intercept	-7.621	4.2609	-1.7885	0.1115	-17.4463
GRE VERBAL	-0.023	0.0448	-0.5123	0.6223	-0.1262
GRE QUANTITATIVE	0.089	0.0597	1.4877	0.1751	-0.0489
GRE WRITING	0.078	0.0757	1.0302	0.3330	-0.0966

Fig. 7.5 Final Spreadsheet for GRE vs. FIRST-YEAR GPA Regression Analysis

Once you have the SUMMARY OUTPUT, you can determine the multiple correlation and the regression equation that is the best-fit line through the data points using GRE VERBAL, GRE QUANTITATIVE, and GRE WRITING as the three predictors, and FIRST-YEAR GPA as the criterion.

Note on the SUMMARY OUTPUT where it says: "Multiple R." This term is correct since this is the term Excel uses for the multiple correlation, which is +0.91. This means, that from these data, the combination of GRE VERBAL, GRE QUANTITATIVE, and GRE WRITING scores together form a very strong positive relationship in predicting FIRST-YEAR GPA.

To find the regression equation, *notice the coefficients at the bottom of the SUMMARY OUTPUT in cells B36 – B 39*:

Intercept: a (this is the y-intercept)	*−7.621*
GRE VERBAL SCORE*: b_1*	*−0.023*
GRE QUANTITATIVE SCORE: b_2	*0.089*
GRE WRITING SCORE: *b_3*	0.078

Since the general form of the multiple regression equation is:

$$Y = a + b_1X_1 + b_2X_2 + b_3X_3 \tag{7.2}$$

we can now write the multiple regression equation for these data:

$$Y = -7.621 - 0.023\,X_1 + 0.089\,X_2 + 0.078X_3$$

7.3 Using the Regression Equation to Predict FIRST-YEAR GPA

Objective: To find the predicted FIRST-YEAR GPA using a GRE VERBAL Score of 158, a GRE QUANTITATIVE Score of 163, and a GRE WRITING Score of 4

Plugging these three numbers into our regression equation gives us:

$$\text{Y} = -7.621 - 0.023(158) + 0.089(163) + 0.078(4)$$

$$\text{Y} = -7.621 - 3.634 + 14.507 + 0.312$$

$$\text{Y} = 3.56 \text{ (since GPA scores are typically measured in two decimals)}$$

If you want to learn more about the theory behind multiple regression, see Keller (2009) and Veney et al. (2009).

7.4 Using Excel to Create a Correlation Matrix in Multiple Regression

The final step in multiple regression is to find the correlation between all of the variables that appear in the regression equation.

In our example, this means that we need to find the correlation between each of the six pairs of variables:

To do this, we need to use Excel to create a "correlation matrix." This matrix summarizes the correlations between all of the variables in the problem.

Objective: To use Excel to create a correlation matrix between the four variables in this example.

To use Excel to do this, use these steps:
Data (top of screen under "Home" at the top left of screen)
Data Analysis
Correlation (scroll *up* to highlight this formula; see Fig. 7.6)

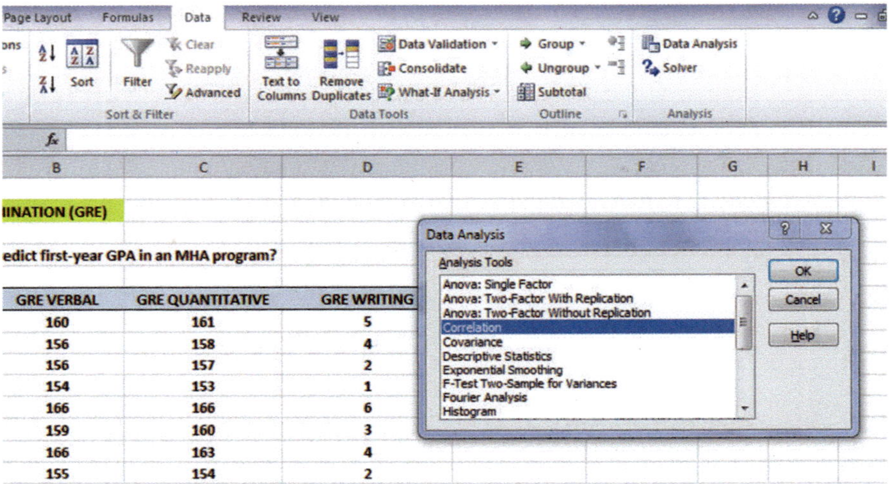

Fig. 7.6 Dialogue Box for GRE vs. FIRST-YEAR GPA Correlations

OK

Input range: A6:D18

(Note that this input range includes the labels at the top of the FOUR variables (FIRST-YEAR GPA, GRE VERBAL, GRE QUANTITATIVE, and GRE WRITING) as well as all of the figures in the original data set).
Grouped by: Columns
Put a check in the box for: Labels in the First Row (since you included the labels at the top of the columns in your input range of data above)
Output range (click on the button to its left, and enter): A42 (see Fig. 7.7)

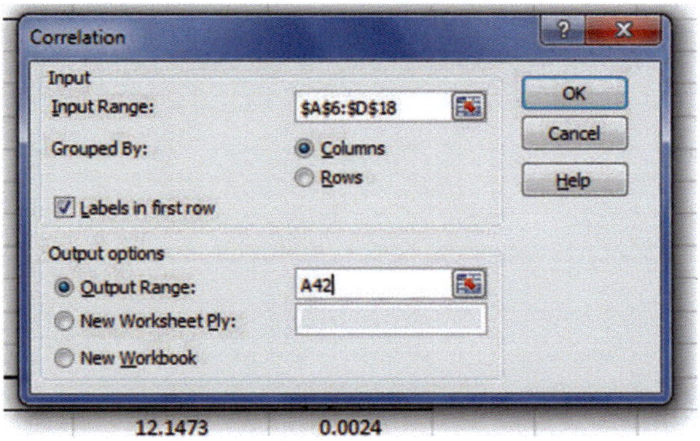

Fig. 7.7 Dialogue Box for Input/Output Range for Correlation Matrix

OK

The resulting correlation matrix appears in A42:E46 (See Fig. 7.8).

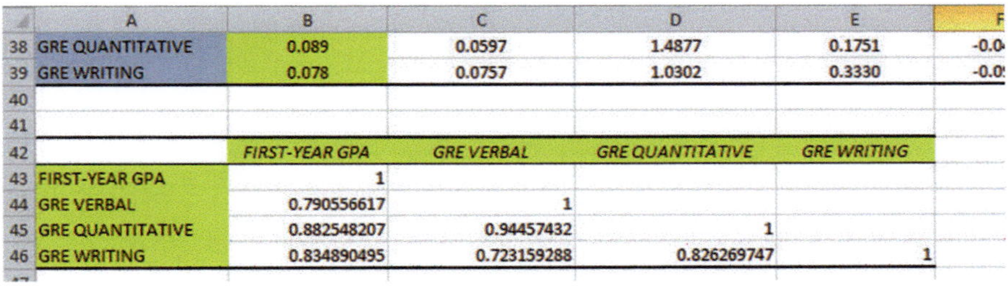

	A	B	C	D	E	F
38	GRE QUANTITATIVE	0.089	0.0597	1.4877	0.1751	-0.0
39	GRE WRITING	0.078	0.0757	1.0302	0.3330	-0.0
40						
41						
42		FIRST-YEAR GPA	GRE VERBAL	GRE QUANTITATIVE	GRE WRITING	
43	FIRST-YEAR GPA	1				
44	GRE VERBAL	0.790556617	1			
45	GRE QUANTITATIVE	0.882548207	0.94457432	1		
46	GRE WRITING	0.834890495	0.723159288	0.826269747	1	

Fig. 7.8 Resulting Correlation Matrix for GRE vs. FIRST-YEAR GPA Data

Next, format all of the numbers in the correlation matrix that are in decimals to two decimals places. And, also, make column D wider so that the GRE QUANTITIVE score label fits inside cell D42.

Re-save this Excel file as: GRE3

The final spreadsheet for these scores appears in Fig. 7.9.

GRADUATE RECORD EXAMINATION (GRE)

How well does the GRE predict first-year GPA in an MHA program?

FIRST-YEAR GPA	GRE VERBAL	GRE QUANTITATIVE	GRE WRITING
3.25	160	161	5
3.42	156	158	4
2.85	156	157	2
2.65	154	153	1
3.65	166	166	6
3.16	159	160	3
3.56	166	163	4
2.35	155	154	2
2.86	153	154	3
2.95	158	157	4
3.15	158	159	4
3.45	160	160	5

SUMMARY OUTPUT

Regression Statistics	
Multiple R	0.91
R Square	0.8200
Adjusted R Square	0.7525
Standard Error	0.1941
Observations	12

ANOVA

	df	*SS*	*MS*	*F*	*Significance F*
Regression	3	1.3730	0.4577	12.1473	0.0024
Residual	8	0.3014	0.0377		
Total	11	1.6744			

	Coefficients	*Standard Error*	*t Stat*	*P-value*	*Lower 95%*
Intercept	-7.621	4.2609	-1.7885	0.1115	-17.4463
GRE VERBAL	-0.023	0.0448	-0.5123	0.6223	-0.1262
GRE QUANTITATIVE	0.089	0.0597	1.4877	0.1751	-0.0489
GRE WRITING	0.078	0.0757	1.0302	0.3330	-0.0966

	FIRST-YEAR GPA	*GRE VERBAL*	*GRE QUANTITATIVE*	*GRE WRITING*
FIRST-YEAR GPA	1			
GRE VERBAL	0.79	1		
GRE QUANTITATIVE	0.88	0.94	1	
GRE WRITING	0.83	0.72	0.83	1

Fig. 7.9 Final Spreadsheet for GRE vs. FIRST-YEAR GPA Regression and the Correlation Matrix

Note that the number "1" along the diagonal of the correlation matrix means that the correlation of each variable with itself is a perfect, positive correlation of 1.0.

Correlation coefficients are always expressed in just two decimal places.

You are now ready to read the correlation between the six pairs of variables:

The correlation between GRE VERBAL and FIRST-YEAR GPA is: +.79
The correlation between GRE QUANTITATIVE and FIRST-YEAR GPA is: +.88
The correlation between GRE WRITING and FIRST-YEAR GPA is: +.83
The correlation between GRE VERBAL and GRE QUANTITATIVE is: +.94
The correlation between GRE VERBAL and GRE WRITING is: +.72
The correlation between GRE QUANTITATIVE and GRE WRITING is: +.83

This means that the best single predictor of FIRST-YEAR GPA is the GRE QUANTITATIVE SCORE with a correlation of +.88. Adding the other two predictor variables, GRE VERBAL and GRE WRITING, improved the prediction by only 0.03 to 0.91, resulting in only a slightly better prediction. GRE QUANTITATIVE scores are an excellent predictor of FIRST-YEAR GPA all by themselves.

If you want to learn more about the correlation matrix, see Levine et al. (2011) and Veney (2003).

7.5 End-of-Chapter Practice Problems

1. Suppose an administrator at a multi-institutional health service organization wants to study the insured population at the organization to determine the relationship between the number of visits to the nearest clinic in the past year and both the age of the patient and the distance from the nearest clinic of the patient's home (measured in miles). Is there a relationship between the age of the patient, the distance to the nearest clinic, and the number of visits to the nearest clinic during the past year?

   You have decided to use a multiple correlation and multiple regression analysis to answer these questions, and to test your Excel skills, you have collected the data of a random sample of 17 patients during the past year. These hypothetical data appear in Fig. 7.10:

RELATIONSHIP BETWEEN VISITS, AGE, AND DISTANCE TO THE NEAREST CLINIC

VISITS	AGE	DISTANCE
5	40	0.3
1	23	7.2
1	18	4.3
7	53	1.5
2	28	6.1
5	25	3.2
5	58	0.2
6	40	2.3
1	25	6.1
8	54	1.3
6	51	1.1
1	20	5.8
3	35	1.4
2	23	5.3
5	51	1.4
5	58	1.1
3	30	2.4

Fig. 7.10 Worksheet Data for Chap. 7: Practice Problem #1

(a) Create an Excel spreadsheet using VISITS as the criterion (Y), and AGE (X_1) and DISTANCE (X_2) as the predictors.
(b) Use Excel's *multiple regression* function to find the relationship between these three variables and place it below the table.
(c) Use number format (two decimal places) for the multiple correlation on the SUMMARY OUTPUT, and use four decimal places for the coefficients in the SUMMARY OUTPUT
(d) Print the table and regression results below the table so that they fit onto one page.
(e) Save this file as: VISITS11

Answer the following questions using your Excel printout:

1. What is the multiple correlation R_{xy} ?
2. What is the y-intercept a?
3. What is the coefficient for AGE b_1?
4. What is the coefficient for DISTANCE b_2?
5. What is the multiple regression equation?
6. Predict the number of visits you would expect for an age of 34 and a distance of 5 miles.

(f) Now, go back to your Excel file and create a *correlation matrix* for these three variables, and place it underneath the SUMMARY OUTPUT.
(g) Re-save this file as: VISITS11
(h) Now, print out *just this correlation matrix* on a separate sheet of paper.

Answer the following questions using your Excel printout. Be sure to include the plus or minus sign for each correlation:

7. What is the correlation between AGE and VISITS?
8. What is the correlation between DISTANCE and VISITS?
9. What is the correlation between DISTANCE and AGE?
10. Discuss which of the two predictors is the better predictor of VISITS.
11. Explain in words how much better the two predictor variables together predict VISITS than the better single predictor by itself.

2. Suppose that you wanted to study the ability of Age, Undergraduate GPA, and SAT Math scores to predict the final grade on a required Bachelor of Social Work (BSW) course in Statistics (100 points possible) that was restricted to seniors in the program. Is there a relationship between the students' age, undergraduate GPA, SAT Math score and the ability of these three predictors to predict the final exam score in this Statistics course? You want to test your Excel skills before you collect the data to answer this question, and you have created the hypothetical data given in Fig. 7.11.

FINAL EXAM RESULTS IN THE REQUIRED STATISTICS COURSE IN THE BSW PROGRAM			
How well do Age, Undergraduate GPA, and SAT Math scores predict Final Exam scores in Statistics?			
FINAL EXAM	AGE	GPA	SAT MATH
92	20	3.62	740
88	19	3.45	720
91	21	3.84	680
85	22	2.85	650
75	24	2.50	610
86	21	3.42	620
84	20	3.15	550
85	19	3.64	580
79	25	3.05	590
73	23	2.95	610
76	24	2.84	630
80	22	3.06	620
79	23	3.10	560

Fig. 7.11 Worksheet Data for Chap. 7: Practice Problem #2

(a) create an Excel spreadsheet using FINAL EXAM as the criterion (Y), and the other variables as the three predictors of this criterion.
(b) Use Excel's *multiple regression* function to find the relationship between these four variables and place it below the table.
(c) Use number format (two decimal places) for the multiple correlation on the Summary Output, and use number format (three decimal places) for the coefficients and all other decimal figures in the Summary Output.
(d) Print the table and regression results below the table so that they fit onto one page.
(e) By hand on this printout, *circle and label:*

(1a) multiple correlation R_{xy}
(2b) coefficients for the y-intercept, AGE, GPA, and SAT MATH.

(f) Save this file as: GPA20

(g) Now, go back to your Excel file and create a correlation matrix for these four variables, and place it underneath the Summary Table. *Change each correlation to just two decimals.* Save this file again as: GPA20
(h) Now, print out *just this correlation matrix in portrait mode* on a separate sheet of paper.

Answer the following questions using your Excel printout:

1. What is the multiple correlation R_{xy}?
2. What is the y-intercept *a*?
3. What is the coefficient for AGE: b_1?

4. What is the coefficient for GPA: b_2?
5. what is the coefficient for SAT MATH: b_3?
6. What is the multiple regression equation?
7. Underneath this regression equation by hand, predict the FINAL EXAM score you would expect for an AGE of 21, a GPA of 3.25, and an SAT MATH score of 650.

Answer the following questions using your Excel printout. Be sure to include the plus or minus sign for each correlation:

8. What is the correlation between AGE and FINAL EXAM?
9. What is the correlation between GPA and FINAL EXAM?
10. What is the correlation between SAT MATH and FINAL EXAM?
11. What is the correlation between AGE and GPA?
12. What is the correlation between GPA and SAT MATH?
13. Discuss which of the three predictors is the best predictor of FINAL EXAM.
14. Explain in words how much better the three predictor variables combined predict FINAL EXAM than the best single predictor by itself.

3. Suppose that you wanted to study the relationship between the number of visits to a health care clinic during the past year by the insured population (i.e., the volume of care provided to the patient) and the ability of the patient to pay for care services (measured by dividing the disposable family income of the patient by the patient's family size) and the distance (to the nearest mile) from the patient's residence to the clinic. For example, is distance negatively correlated with the number of visits?

   You have decided to use a multiple correlation and multiple regression analysis, and to test your Excel skills, you have collected the data of a random sample of 15 patients who were treated for the same condition during the past year.

   These hypothetical data appear in Fig. 7.12.

INSURED POPULATION		
VISITS	INCOME ($000)*	DISTANCE (nearest mile)
3	16	8
2	13	10
1	14	12
4	9	2
1	6	12
2	10	11
4	24	3
2	9	12
2	16	10
6	32	4
5	39	3
6	38	2
3	9	5
4	26	5
5	34	2

* INCOME = DISPOSABLE FAMILY INCOME DIVIDED BY FAMILY SIZE

Fig. 7.12 Worksheet Data for Chap. 7: Practice Problem #3

(a) create an Excel spreadsheet using the number of visits as the criterion and the other two variables as the predictors.
(b) Use Excel's *multiple regression* function to find the relationship between these three variables and place the SUMMARY OUTPUT below the table.
(c) Use number format (two decimal places) for the multiple correlation on the Summary Output, and use number format (three decimal places) for the coefficients in the summary output and for all other decimal figures in the SUMMARY OUTPUT.
(d) Save the file as: VISITS21
(e) Print the table and regression results below the table so that they fit onto one page.

Answer the following questions using your Excel printout:

1. What is multiple correlation R_{xy}?
2. What is the y-intercept a?
3. What is the coefficient for INCOME b_1?
4. What is the coefficient for DISTANCE b_2?
5. What is the multiple regression equation?
6. Predict the number of visits you would expect for an adjusted INCOME of $26,000 and a distance of 4 miles.

(f) Now, go back to your Excel file and create a correlation matrix for these three variables, and place it underneath the SUMMARY OUTPUT on your spreadsheet.

(g) Re-save this file as: VISITS21
(h) Now, print out *just this correlation matrix* on a separate sheet of paper.

Answer the following questions using your Excel printout. Be sure to include the plus or minus sign for each correlation:

7. What is the correlation between INCOME and VISITS?
8. What is the correlation between DISTANCE and VISITS?
9. What is the correlation between DISTANCE and INCOME?
10. Discuss which of the two predictors is the better predictor of VISITS.
11. Explain in words how much better the two predictor variables combined predict VISITS than the better single predictor by itself.

References

Keller G. Statistics for management and economics. 8th ed. Mason: South-Western Cengage Learning; 2009.

Levine D, Stephan D, Krehbiel T, Berenson M. Statistics for managers using Microsoft Excel. 6th ed. Boston: Pearson Prentice Hall; 2011.

Veney J E. Statistics for health policy and administration using Microsoft Excel. San Francisco: Jossey-Bass; 2003

Veney J E, Kros J F, Rosenthal D A. Statistics for health care professionals: working with Excel. 2nd ed. San Francisco: Jossey-Bass; 2009.

Chapter 8
One-Way Analysis of Variance (ANOVA)

So far in this 2016 Excel Guide, you have learned how to use a one-group t-test to compare the sample mean to the population mean, and a two-group t-test to test for the difference between two sample means. *But what should you do when you have more than two groups and you want to determine if there is a significant difference between the means of these groups?*

The answer to this question is: *Analysis of Variance (ANOVA).*

The ANOVA test allows you to test for the difference between the means when you have *three or more groups* in your research study. The null hypothesis is that all of the population means are equal. The research hypothesis is that at least two of the population means are significantly different from one another. To conduct an ANOVA test, you need to assume both that the populations are normally distributed and also that they have equal standard deviations.

Important note: In order to do One-way Analysis of Variance, you need to have installed the "Data Analysis Toolpak" that was described in Chap. 6 (see Sect. 6.5.1). If you did not install this, you need to do that now!

Let's suppose you are working as a social work researcher in a health care system and want to compare the diagnostic time required for an initial new patient visit at each of the three clinics your company operates (Clinic A, Clinic B, and Clinic C). Assume that you have recorded the number of minutes (to the nearest minute) to complete a new patient diagnostic visit at each of the three clinics by taking a random sample of initial visitors during the past six months. The hypothetical results are given in Fig. 8.1.

T.J. Quirk, S. Cummings, *Excel 2016 for Social Work Statistics*, Excel for Statistics,
DOI 10.1007/978-3-319-66221-3_8

Fig. 8.1 Worksheet Data for Initial Visits (Practical Example)

DIAGNOSTIC TIME OF INITIAL VISIT

(data are in minutes)

Clinic A	Clinic B	Clinic C
23	16	14
37	23	22
26	21	21
24	18	23
25	17	18
29	22	19
30	19	20
35	16	20
32		15
31		

You have been asked to analyze the data to determine if there was any significant difference in diagnostic time between the three clinics. Note that it is not necessary for each clinic to see the same number of patients or to have the same sample size in order for ANOVA to be used on the data. Statisticians delight in this fact by stating that: "ANOVA is a very robust test." (Statisticians love that term!)

Create an Excel spreadsheet for these data in this way:

A4: DIAGNOSTIC TIME OF INITIAL VISIT
A6: (data are in minutes)
B8: Clinic A
C8: Clinic B
D8: Clinic C
B9: 23

Enter the other information into your spreadsheet table. When you have finished entering these data, the last cell on the left should have 31 in cell B18, and the last cell on the right should have 15 in cell D17. Center the numbers in each of the columns. Use number format (zero decimals) for all numbers.

Important note: Be sure to double-check all of your figures in the table to make sure that they are exactly correct or you will not be able to obtain the correct answer for this problem!

Save this file as: CLINIC6

8.1 Using Excel to Perform a One-Way Analysis of Variance (ANOVA)

Objective: To use Excel to perform a one-way ANOVA test.

You are now ready to perform an ANOVA test on these data using the following steps:

Data (at top of screen)
Data Analysis (far right at top of screen)
Anova: Single Factor (*scroll up to this formula and highlight it*; see Fig. 8.2)

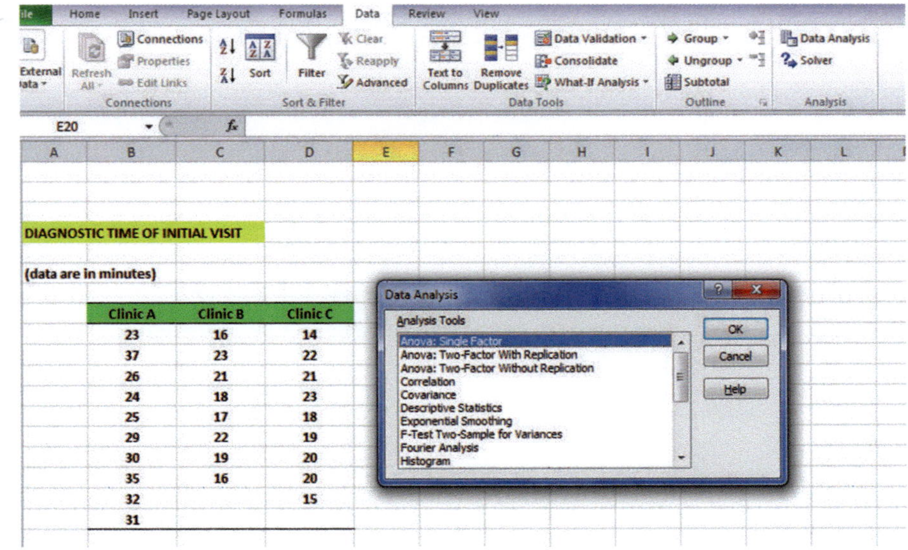

Fig. 8.2 Dialog Box for Data Analysis: ANOVA Single Factor

OK

Input range: B8:D18 (note that you have included in this range the column titles that are in row 8)

Important note: Whenever the data set has a different sample size in the groups being compared, the INPUT RANGE that you define must start at the column title of the first group on the left and go to the last column on the right to the lowest row that has a figure in it in the entire data matrix so that the INPUT RANGE has the "shape" of a rectangle when you highlight it. Since Clinic A has 31 in cell B18, your "rectangle" must include row 18!

Grouped by: Columns
Put a check mark in: Labels in First Row
Output range (click on the button to its left): A22 (see Fig. 8.3)

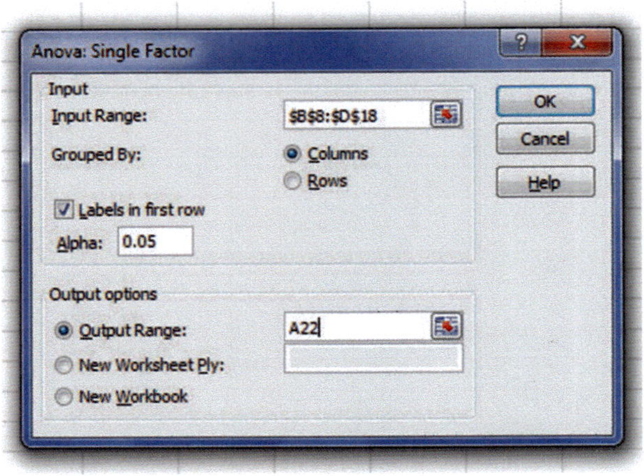

Fig. 8.3 Dialog Box for ANOVA: Single Factor Input/Output Range

OK

Center all of the numbers in the ANOVA table, and round off all numbers that are decimals to two decimal places.

Save this file as: CLINIC6A

You should have generated the table given in Fig. 8.4.

	A	B	C	D	E	F	G
14		29	22	19			
15		30	19	20			
16		35	16	20			
17		32		15			
18		31					
19							
20							
21							
22	Anova: Single Factor						
23							
24	SUMMARY						
25	*Groups*	*Count*	*Sum*	*Average*	*Variance*		
26	Clinic A	10	292	29.20	22.18		
27	Clinic B	8	152	19.00	7.43		
28	Clinic C	9	172	19.11	9.11		
29							
30							
31	ANOVA						
32	*Source of Variation*	*SS*	*df*	*MS*	*F*	*P-value*	*F crit*
33	Between Groups	647.59	2	323.79	23.95	0.00	3.40
34	Within Groups	324.49	24	13.52			
35							
36	Total	972.07	26				
37							

Fig. 8.4 ANOVA Results for the initial visits

Print out both the data table and the ANOVA summary table so that all of this information fits onto one page. (Hint: Set the Page Layout/Fit to Scale to *85% size*).

As a check on your analysis, you should have the following in these cells:

A22: Anova: Single Factor
D26: 29.20
D33: 323.79
E33: 23.95
G33: 3.40

Now, let's discuss how you should interpret this table:

8.2 How to Interpret the ANOVA Table Correctly

Objective: To interpret the ANOVA table correctly

ANOVA allows you to test for the differences between means when you have three or more groups of data. This ANOVA test is called the F-test statistic, and is typically identified with the letter: F.

The formula for the F-test is this:

F = Mean Square between groups (MS_b) divided by Mean Square within groups (MS_w)

$$F = MS_b / MS_w \tag{8.1}$$

The derivation and explanation of this formula is beyond the scope of this *Excel Guide*. In this *Excel Guide*, we are attempting to teach you *how to use Excel to conduct statistical tests*, and we are not attempting to teach you the statistical theory that is behind the ANOVA formulas. For a detailed explanation of ANOVA, see Randolph and Myers (2013) and Veney et al. (2003).

Note that cell D33 contains $MS_b = 323.79$, while cell D34 contains $MS_w = 13.52$.

When you divide these two figures using their cell references in Excel, you get an answer for the F-test of 23.95, which is in cell E33. (Remember, Excel is more accurate than your calculator!) Let's discuss the meaning of the figure: $F = 23.95$.

In order to determine whether this figure for F of 23.95 indicates a significant difference between the means of the three groups, the first step is to write out the null hypothesis and the research hypothesis for the time required to conduct initial visits for each of the three clinics.

In our initial visit comparisons, the null hypothesis states that the population means of the three groups are equal, while the research hypothesis states that the population means of the three groups are not equal, and that there is, therefore, a significant difference between the population means of the three groups. Which of these two hypotheses should you accept based on the ANOVA results?

8.3 Using the Decision Rule for the ANOVA F-Test

To state the hypotheses, let's refer to Clinic A as Group 1, Clinic B as Group 2, and Clinic C as Group 3. The hypotheses would then be:

$H_0: \mu_1 = \mu_2 = \mu_3$
$H_1: \mu_1 \neq \mu_2 \neq \mu_3$

The answer to this question is analogous to the decision rule used in this book for both the one-group t-test and the two-group t-test. You will recall that this rule (See Sects. 4.1.6 and 5.1.8) was:

If the absolute value of t is less than the critical t, you accept the null hypothesis.

or

If the absolute value of t is greater than the critical t, you reject the null hypothesis, and accept the research hypothesis.

Now, here is the decision rule for ANOVA:

Objective: To learn the decision rule for the ANOVA F-test

The decision rule for the ANOVA F-test is the following:

If the value for F is less than the critical F-value, accept the null hypothesis.

or

If the value of F is greater than the critical F-value, reject the null hypothesis, and accept the research hypothesis.

Note that Excel tells you the critical F-value in cell G33: 3.40
Therefore, our decision rule for the initial visits AVOVA test is this:

Since the value of F of 23.95 is greater than the critical F-value of 3.40, we reject the null hypothesis and accept the research hypothesis.

Therefore, our conclusion, in plain English, is:

There was a significant difference between the number of minutes required for the initial diagnostic visit between the three clinics.

Note that it is not necessary to take the absolute value of F of 23.95. The F-value can never be less than one, and so it can never be a negative value which requires us to take its absolute value in order to treat it as a positive value.
It is important to note that ANOVA tells us that there was a significant difference between the population means of the three groups, *but it does not tell us which pairs of groups were significantly different from each other.*

8.4 Testing for the Difference Between Two Groups Using the ANOVA t-Test

To answer that question, we need to do a different test called the ANOVA t-test.

Objective: To test the difference between the means of two groups using an ANOVA t-test when the ANOVA F-test results indicate a significant difference between the population means.

Since we have three groups of data (one group for each of the three clinics), we would have to perform three separate ANOVA t-tests to determine which pairs of groups were significantly different. This requires that we would have to perform a separate ANOVA t-test for the following pairs of groups:

1. Clinic A vs. Clinic B
2. Clinic A vs. Clinic C
3. Clinic B vs. Clinic C

We will do just one of these pairs of tests, Clinic A vs. Clinic C, to illustrate the way to perform an ANOVA t-test comparing these two clinics. The ANOVA t-test for the other two pairs of groups would be done in the same way.

8.4.1 Comparing Clinic A vs. Clinic C in Time Required to Conduct an Initial Visit Using the ANOVA t-Test

Objective: To compare Clinic A vs. Clinic C in minutes required for the initial diagnostic visit using the ANOVA t-test.

The first step is to write out the null hypothesis and the research hypothesis for these two clinics.

For the ANOVA t-test, the null hypothesis is that the population means of the two groups are equal, while the research hypothesis is that the population means of the two groups are not equal (i.e., there is a significant difference between these two means). Since we are comparing Clinic A (Group 1) vs. Clinic C (Group 3), these hypotheses would be:

$H_0: \mu_1 = \mu_3$
$H_1: \mu_1 \neq \mu_3$

For Group 1 vs. Group 3, the formula for the ANOVA t-test is:

$$ANOVA\ t = \frac{\bar{X}_1 - \bar{X}_2}{s.e._{ANOVA}} \tag{8.2}$$

where

$$s.e._{ANOVA} = \sqrt{MS_w \left(\frac{1}{n_1} + \frac{1}{n_2} \right)} \tag{8.3}$$

Important note: Formula 8.3 uses n_1 and n_2, but since we are comparing Group 1 and Group 3, you should use n_1 and n_3 in your use of this formula.

The steps involved in computing this ANOVA t-test are:

1. Find the difference of the sample means for the two groups: (29.20 − 19.11 = 10.09).
2. Find $1/n_1 + 1/n_3$ (since both groups have a different number of visitors in them, this becomes: 1/10 + 1/9 = 0.10 + 0.11 = 0.21
3. Multiply MS_w times the answer for step 2: (13.52 × 0.21 = 2.84)
4. Take the square root of step 3: SQRT (2.84) = 1.68
5. Divide Step 1 by Step 4 to find the ANOVA t: (10.09/1.68 = 6.00)

Note: Since Excel computes all calculations to 16 decimal places, when you use Excel for the above computations, your answer will be 5.97 in two decimal places. Excel's answer will be much more accurate because it always uses 16 decimal places in its computations.

Now, what do we do with this ANOVA t-test result of 6.00? In order to interpret this value of 6.00 correctly, we need to determine the critical value of t for the ANOVA t-test. To do that, we need to find the degrees of freedom for the ANOVA t-test as follows:

8.4.1.1 Finding the Degrees of Freedom for the ANOVA t-Test

Objective: To find the degrees of freedom for the ANOVA t-test.

The degrees of freedom (df) for the ANOVA t-test is found as follows:

df = take the total sample size of all of the groups and subtract the number of groups in your study ($n_{TOTAL} - k$ where k = the number of groups)

In our example, the total sample size of the three groups is 27 since there are 10 visitors in Group 1, 8 visitors in Group 2, and 9 visitors in Group 3, and since there are three groups, 27–3 gives a degrees of freedom for the ANOVA t-test of 24.

If you look up df = 24 in the t-table in Appendix E in the degrees of freedom column (df), which is the *second column on the left of this table*, you will find that the critical t-value is 2.064.

Important note: Be sure to use the degrees of freedom column (df) in Appendix E for the ANOVA t-test critical t value

8.4.1.2 Stating the Decision Rule for the ANOVA t-Test

Objective: To learn the decision rule for the ANOVA t-test

Interpreting the result of the ANOVA t-test follows the same decision rule that we used for both the one-group t-test (see Sect. 4.1.6) and the two-group t-test (see Sect. 5.1.8):

If the absolute value of t is less than the critical value of t, we accept the null hypothesis.

or

If the absolute value of t is greater than the critical value of t, we reject the null hypothesis and accept the research hypothesis.

Since we are using a type of t-test, we need to take the absolute value of t. Since the absolute value of 6.00 is greater than the critical t-value of 2.064, we reject the null hypothesis (that the population means of the two groups are equal) and accept the research hypothesis (that the population means of the two groups are significantly different from one another).

This means that our conclusion, in plain English, is as follows:

The average initial diagnostic visit at Clinic A was significantly longer than the average initial diagnostic visit at Clinic C (29 minutes vs. 19 minutes).

8.4.1.3 Performing an ANOVA t-Test Using Excel Commands

Now, let's do these calculations for the ANOVA t-test using Excel with the file you created earlier in this chapter: CLINIC6A

A39: Clinic A vs. Clinic C
A41: 1/10 + 1/9
A43: s.e. ANOVA
A45: ANOVA t-test
B41: =(1/10 + 1/9) (no spaces between symbols)
B43: =SQRT(D34*B41) (no spaces between symbols)
B45: =(D26 – D28)/B43 (no spaces between symbols)

You should now have the following results in these cells when you round off all these figures in the ANOVA t-test to two decimal points.

B41: 0.21
B43: 1.69
B45: 5.97

Save this final result under the file name: CLINIC7

Print out the resulting spreadsheet so that it fits onto one page like Fig. 8.5 (Hint: Reduce the Page Layout/Scale to Fit to *85%*).

DIAGNOSTIC TIME OF INITIAL VISIT			
(data are in minutes)			
	Clinic A	Clinic B	Clinic C
	23	16	14
	37	23	22
	26	21	21
	24	18	23
	25	17	18
	29	22	19
	30	19	20
	35	16	20
	32		15
	31		

Anova: Single Factor

SUMMARY

Groups	Count	Sum	Average	Variance
Clinic A	10	292	29.20	22.18
Clinic B	8	152	19.00	7.43
Clinic C	9	172	19.11	9.11

ANOVA

Source of Variation	SS	df	MS	F	P-value	F crit
Between Groups	647.59	2	323.79	23.95	0.00	3.40
Within Groups	324.49	24	13.52			
Total	972.07	26				

Clinic A vs. Clinic C	
1/10 + 1/9	0.21
s.e. ANOVA	1.69
ANOVA t-test	5.97

Fig. 8.5 Final Spreadsheet of Initial Visit for Clinic A vs. Clinic C

For a more detailed explanation of the ANOVA t-test, see Scott and Mazhindu (2005) and Black (2010).

Important note: You are only allowed to perform an ANOVA t-test comparing the means of two groups when the F-test produces a significant difference between the means of all of the groups in your study.

It is improper to do any ANOVA t-test when the value of F is less than the critical value of F. Whenever F is less than the critical F, this means that there was no difference between the means of the groups, and, therefore, any test conducted to see if there is a difference between the means of these two groups would capitalize on chance differences between the two groups.

8.5 End-of-Chapter Practice Problems

1. When universities in the USA want to hire qualified faculty, they typically advertise for the position on a Web site for professional organizations that include job openings on the Web site so that members of the organizations can become informed about possible job matches in their career search. If a university wants to hire a new qualified faculty member to teach Social Work, there are three popular Web sites that provide this job listing: (1) The National Association of Social Workers (NASW), (2) The Council on Social Work Education (CSWE), and (3) The Chronicle of Higher Education. Suppose that a university wants to determine if there was a difference in applications received from these three Web sites when the past eight professors of Social Work were hired by that university. The hypothetical data for this study are given in Fig. 8.6.

Fig. 8.6 Worksheet Data for Chap. 8: Practice Problem #1

SOURCE OF SOCIAL WORK TEACHING APPLICATIONS

NUMBER OF APPLICATIONS

CHRONICLE	NASW	CSWE
85	68	86
64	64	89
92	65	102
54	62	116
68	63	101
67	61	98
55	60	95
82	59	94

(a) Enter these data on an Excel spreadsheet.
(b) Perform a *one-way ANOVA test* on these data, and show the resulting ANOVA table *underneath* the input data for the three Web sites.
(c) If the F-value in the ANOVA table is significant, create an Excel formula to compute the ANOVA t-test comparing the average applications for NASW

against the average applications for CSWE, and show the results below the ANOVA table on the spreadsheet (put the standard error and the ANOVA t-test value on separate lines of your spreadsheet, and use two decimal places for each value)

(d) Print out the resulting spreadsheet so that all of the information fits onto one page

(e) Save the spreadsheet as: JOB12

Now, write the answers to the following questions using your Excel printout:

1. What are the null hypothesis and the research hypothesis for the ANOVA F-test?
2. What is MS_b on your Excel printout?
3. What is MS_w on your Excel printout?
4. Compute $F = MS_b/MS_w$ using your calculator.
5. What is the critical value of F on your Excel printout?
6. What is the result of the ANOVA F-test?
7. What is the conclusion of the ANOVA F-test in plain English?
8. If the ANOVA F-test produced a significant difference between the three Web sites in the number of job applications received for a Social Work opening, what is the null hypothesis and the research hypothesis for the ANOVA t-test comparing NASW versus CSWE?
9. What is the mean (average) number of applications for NASW on your Excel printout?
10. What is the mean (average) number of applications for CSWE on your Excel printout?
11. What are the degrees of freedom (df) for the ANOVA t-test comparing NASW versus CSWE?
12. What is the critical t value for this ANOVA t-test in Appendix E for these degrees of freedom?
13. Compute the $s.e._{ANOVA}$ using your calculator for NASW versus CSWE.
14. Compute the ANOVA t-test value comparing NASW versus CSWE using your calculator.
15. What is the result of the ANOVA t-test comparing NASW versus CSWE?
16. What is the conclusion of the ANOVA t-test comparing NASW versus CSWE in plain English?

Note: Since there are three Web sites and they comprise three pairs of Web sites between them, you need to do three ANOVA t-tests to determine what the significant differences are between the three Web sites in job applications received. Since you have just completed the ANOVA t-test comparing NASW versus CSWE, you would also need to do the ANOVA t-test comparing:

CHRONICLE versus NASW
CHRONICLE versus CSWE

in order to write a conclusion summarizing these three ANOVA t-tests overall.

2. In a multi-institutional arrangement, the delay in transferring inpatients to an alternate source of care after hospitalization is an important factor. If you measure "delay" by the number of days between the date when a patient was ready for transfer and the date on which the patient was transferred to a nursing home, you can compare the hospitals in your organization in terms of their days of delay to effect this transfer. Suppose that you decide to take a random sample of inpatients who were transferred from the hospital to a nursing home over the past six months from each of the four hospitals in your system.

   Note that each hospital can have a different sample size of inpatients in order for ANOVA to be used on the data. Statisticians delight in this fact by stating that: "ANOVA is a very robust test." (Statisticians love that term!)

   Suppose that your random sample produces the hypothetical data given in Fig. 8.7.

Fig. 8.7 Worksheet Data for Chap. 8: Practice Problem #2

NUMBER OF DAYS UNTIL TRANSFER TO A NURSING HOME

HOSPITAL			
A	B	C	D
9	5	15	12
11	9	18	14
12	8	16	16
10	7	17	18
12	6	19	17
11	5	21	13
13	7	22	17
9	9	19	16
14	10		15
10			14
13			

   (a) Enter these data on an Excel spreadsheet.
   (b) Perform a *one-way ANOVA test* on these data, and show the resulting ANOVA table *underneath* the input data for the four hospitals. Round off all decimal figures to two decimal places, and center all numbers in the ANOVA table.
   (c) If the F-value in the ANOVA table is significant, create an Excel formula to compute the ANOVA t-test comparing the number of days until transfer for HOSPITAL B against the number of days until transfer for HOSPITAL C, and show the results below the ANOVA table on the spreadsheet (put the standard error and the ANOVA t-test value on separate lines of your spreadsheet, and use two decimal places for each value)

(d) Print out the resulting spreadsheet so that all of the information fits onto one page
(e) Save the spreadsheet as: DAYS3

Now, write the answers to the following questions using your Excel printout:

1. What are the null hypothesis and the research hypothesis for the ANOVA F-test?
2. What is MS_b on your Excel printout?
3. What is MS_w on your Excel printout?
4. Compute $F = MS_b/MS_w$ using your calculator.
5. What is the critical value of F on your Excel printout?
6. What is the result of the ANOVA F-test?
7. What is the conclusion of the ANOVA F-test in plain English?
8. If the ANOVA F-test produced a significant difference between the four hospitals in the days until transfer, what is the null hypothesis and the research hypothesis for the ANOVA t-test comparing HOSPITAL B versus HOSPITAL C?
9. What is the mean (average) number of days until transfer for HOSPITAL B on your Excel printout?
10. What is the mean (average) number of days until transfer for HOSPITAL C on your Excel printout?
11. What are the degrees of freedom (df) for the ANOVA t-test comparing HOSPITAL B versus HOSPITAL C?
12. What is the critical t value for this ANOVA t-test in Appendix E for these degrees of freedom?
13. Compute the $s.e._{ANOVA}$ using Excel for HOSPITAL B versus HOSPITAL C.
14. Compute the ANOVA t-test value comparing HOSPITAL B versus HOSPITAL C using Excel.
15. What is the result of the ANOVA t-test comparing HOSPITAL B versus HOSPITAL C?
16. What is the conclusion of the ANOVA t-test comparing HOSPITAL B versus HOSPITAL C in plain English?

3. Length of stay (LOS) in a health care facility is an important factor in profitability. Suppose that you work for a multi-institutional health care system that includes five health care facilities and you want to compare them on their LOS data. Suppose, further, that you have taken a random sample of inpatients from each of these facilities who have stayed in these facilities during the past 90 days. Recall that ANOVA allows the sample sizes of the groups to be different. The hypothetical data for this study are given in Fig. 8.8.

Fig. 8.8 Worksheet Data for Chap. 8: Practice Problem #3

LENGTH OF STAY (LOS)				
HEALTH CARE FACILITY				
A	B	C	D	E
3	2	3	7	5
4	8	5	11	9
5	4	9	12	6
4	6	6	9	8
5	7	7	8	7
3	3	8	6	6
2	5	4	7	5
4	8	11	10	9
5	9	12	12	7
4	7	10		4
3		11		6
		9		8
				9

(a) Enter these data on an Excel spreadsheet.
(b) Perform a *one-way ANOVA test* on these data, and show the resulting ANOVA table *underneath* the input data for the five types of health care facilities.
(c) If the F-value in the ANOVA table is significant, create an Excel formula to compute the ANOVA t-test comparing the average LOS for FACILITY B against the average LOS for FACILITY E, and show the results below the ANOVA table on the spreadsheet (put the standard error and the ANOVA t-test value on separate lines of your spreadsheet, and use two decimal places for each value)
(d) Print out the resulting spreadsheet so that all of the information fits onto one page
(e) Save the spreadsheet as: STAY3

Now, write the answers to the following questions using your Excel printout:

1. What are the null hypothesis and the research hypothesis for the ANOVA F-test?
2. What is MS_b on your Excel printout?
3. What is MS_w on your Excel printout?
4. Compute $F = MS_b/MS_w$ using your calculator.
5. What is the critical value of F on your Excel printout?
6. What is the result of the ANOVA F-test?
7. What is the conclusion of the ANOVA F-test in plain English?
8. If the ANOVA F-test produced a significant difference between the five types of health care facilities in their LOS, what is the null hypothesis and

the research hypothesis for the ANOVA t-test comparing FACILITY B versus FACILITY E?

9. What is the mean (average) LOS for FACILITY B on your Excel printout?
10. What is the mean (average) LOS for FACILITY E on your Excel printout?
11. What are the degrees of freedom (df) for the ANOVA t-test comparing FACILITY B versus FACILITY E?
12. What is the critical t value for this ANOVA t-test in Appendix E for these degrees of freedom?
13. Compute the $s.e._{ANOVA}$ using your calculator for FACILITY B versus FACILITY E.
14. Compute the ANOVA t-test value comparing FACILITY B versus FACILITY E using your calculator.
15. What is the result of the ANOVA t-test comparing FACILITY B versus FACILITY E?
16. What is the conclusion of the ANOVA t-test comparing FACILITY B versus FACILITY E in plain English?

References

Black K. Business statistics: for contemporary decision making. 6th ed. Hoboken: John Wiley & Sons, Inc.; 2010.

Randolph K, Myers L. Basic statistics in multivariate analysis. New York: Oxford University Press; 2013.

Scott I, Mazhindu D. Statistics for health care professionals: an introduction. Thousand Oaks: Sage; 2005.

Veney J E, Kros J F, Rosenthal D A. Statistics for health care professionals: working with Excel. 2nd ed. San Francisco: Jossey-Bass; 2003.

Appendices

Appendix A: Answers to End-of-Chapter Practice Problems

T.J. Quirk, S. Cummings, *Excel 2016 for Social Work Statistics*, Excel for Statistics,
DOI 10.1007/978-3-319-66221-3

Chapter 1: Practice Problem #1 Answer (see Fig. A.1)

RESIDENTS IN A HOMELESS SHELTER

No. of Nights Spent on the Street Last Month

Nights		
3		
2	n	13
1		
5		
6	Mean	3.54
4		
3		
2	STDEV	1.85
7		
4		
3	s.d.	0.51
5		
1		

Fig. A.1 Answer to Chap. 1: Practice Problem #1

Chapter 1: Practice Problem #2 Answer (see Fig. A.2)

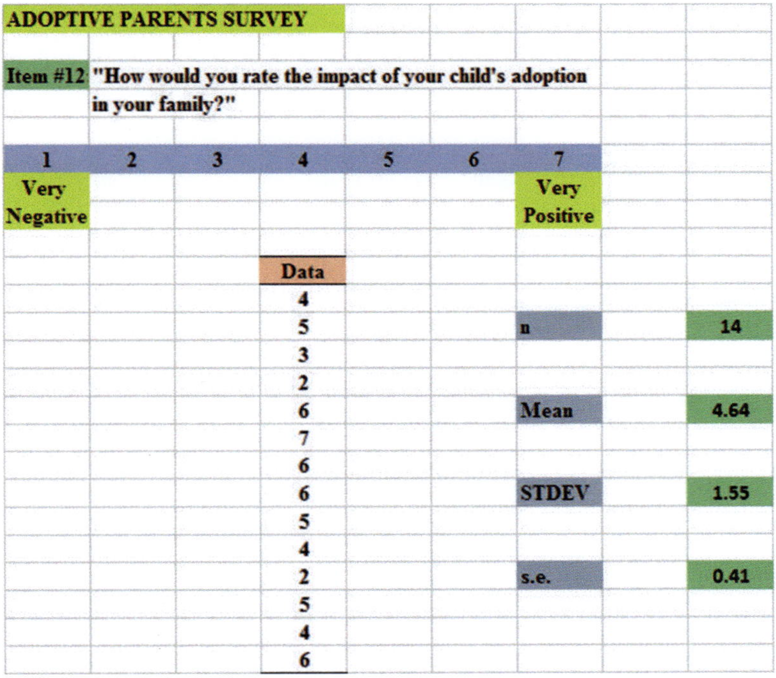

Fig. A.2 Answer to Chap. 1: Practice Problem #2

Chapter 1: Practice Problem #3 Answer (see Fig. A.3)

Fig. A.3 Answer to Chap. 1: Practice Problem #3

MENTAL HEALTH RESPITE CARE FACILITY		
AGE OF GUESTS		
23		
26	n	15
24		
28		
31	Mean	26.600
33		
19		
25	STDEV	3.481
26		
28		
29	s.e.	0.899
30		
27		
24		
26		

Chapter 2: Practice Problem #1 Answer (see Fig. A.4)

FRAME NUMBERS	Duplicate frame numbers	RANDOM NO.
1	7	0.808
2	50	0.817
3	23	0.068
4	13	0.953
5	6	0.274
6	14	0.716
7	60	0.969
8	37	0.515
9	61	0.749
10	33	0.070
11	43	0.345
12	4	0.011
13	8	0.129
14	5	0.379
15	59	0.465
16	39	0.839
17	63	0.863
18	35	0.970
19	49	0.856
20	1	0.742
21	57	0.653
22	12	0.089
23	[illegible]	[illegible]
	[illegible]	0.5[illegible]
56	19	0.737
57	45	0.891
58	21	0.580
59	38	0.003
60	17	0.684
61	11	0.249
62	42	0.563
63	54	0.094

Fig. A.4 Answer to Chap. 2: Practice Problem #1

Chapter 2: Practice Problem #2 Answer (see Fig. A.5)

Fig. A.5 Answer to Chap. 2: Practice Problem #2

FRAME NO.	Duplicate frame no.	Random number
1	58	0.113
2	50	0.716
3	43	0.441
4	42	0.688
5	86	0.702
6	24	0.974
7	22	0.551
8	11	0.815
9	104	0.616
10	105	0.351
11	61	0.091
12	41	0.842
13	79	0.196
14	93	0.066
15	85	0.849
16	54	0.557
17	16	0.968
18	77	0.313
19	15	0.434
20	112	0.984
[illegible]	28	[illegible]
[illegible]	[illegible]	0.786
98	53	0.395
99	40	0.454
100	96	0.534
101	48	0.334
102	108	0.752
103	109	0.694
104	33	0.464
105	3	0.933
106	90	0.577
107	110	0.844
108	62	0.769
109	88	0.719
110	60	0.180
111	98	0.628
112	94	0.440
113	59	0.486
114	67	0.059

Chapter 2: Practice Problem #3 Answer (see Fig. A.6)

FRAME NUMBERS	Duplicate frame numbers	Random number
1	58	0.002
2	7	0.522
3	37	0.945
4	49	0.792
5	26	0.425
6	65	0.131
7	48	0.507
8	63	0.011
9	15	0.659
10	25	0.765
11	21	0.663
12	36	0.247
13	43	0.102
14	11	0.038
15	10	0.644
16	39	0.293
17	72	0.137
18	59	0.508
19	16	0.715
20	54	0.389
21	52	0.987
22	3	0.457
23	[illegible]	[illegible]
[illegible]	6	0.74[illegible]
59	33	0.828
60	31	0.937
61	35	0.697
62	51	0.120
63	62	0.512
64	41	0.027
65	47	0.390
66	14	0.276
67	13	0.683
68	38	0.590
69	17	0.527
70	57	0.666
71	60	0.701
72	9	0.586
73	20	0.822
74	18	0.157
75	5	0.766

Fig. A.6 Answer to Chap. 2: Practice Problem #3

Chapter 3: Practice Problem #1 Answer (see Fig. A.7)

SELF-ESTEEM MEASURE OF HIGH SCHOOL SENIORS

DRUG TREATMENT PROGRAM OUTCOME MEASURE

Item #10: **"I take a positive attitude toward myself."**

4	3	2	1
Strongly Agree	Agree	Disagree	Strongly Disagree

RATING		
4		
2	Null hypothesis:	μ = 2.5
3		
2	Research hypothesis:	$\mu \neq$ 2.5
4		
3		
3	n	15
4		
4	Mean	3.2
1		
3	STDEV	0.9
4		
4	s.e.	0.2
3		
4	95% confidence level	

Lower limit	2.7
Upper limit	3.7

Draw a picture of the confidence interval

----------2.5----- ----2.7----------- -----3.2---------------- -----3.7----

Ref Value	lower limit	Mean	upper limit

Result: Since the reference value is outside of the confidence interval, we reject the null hypothesis and accept the research hypothesis.

Conclusion:: High school seniors who have completed the drug treatment program significantly agreed that they take a positive attitude toward themselves.

Fig. A.7 Answer to Chap. 3: Practice Problem #1

Chapter 3: Practice Problem #2 Answer (see Fig. A.8)

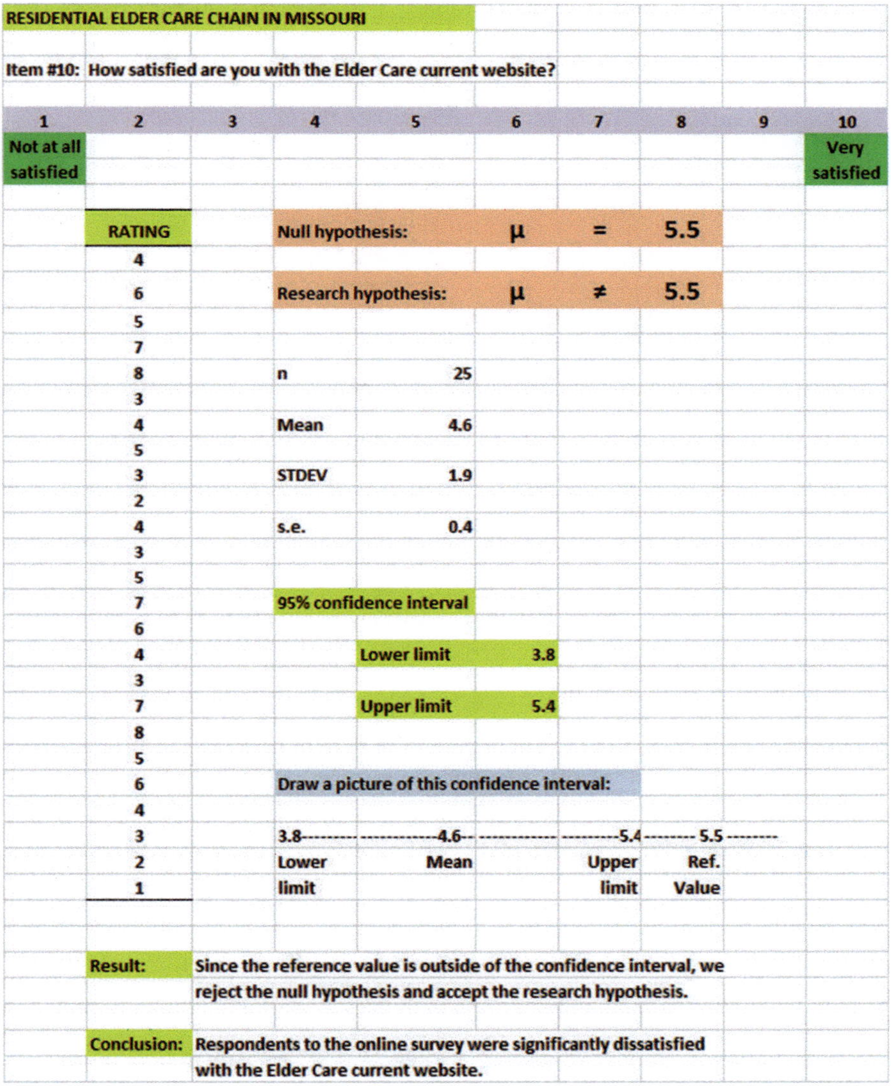

RESIDENTIAL ELDER CARE CHAIN IN MISSOURI									
Item #10:	How satisfied are you with the Elder Care current website?								
1	2	3	4	5	6	7	8	9	10
Not at all satisfied									Very satisfied
	RATING		Null hypothesis:		μ	=	5.5		
	4								
	6		Research hypothesis:		μ	≠	5.5		
	5								
	7								
	8		n	25					
	3								
	4		Mean	4.6					
	5								
	3		STDEV	1.9					
	2								
	4		s.e.	0.4					
	3								
	5								
	7		95% confidence interval						
	6								
	4			Lower limit	3.8				
	3								
	7			Upper limit	5.4				
	8								
	5								
	6		Draw a picture of this confidence interval:						
	4								
	3		3.8---------	------------4.6--	------------	---------5.4	-------- 5.5 --------		
	2		Lower	Mean		Upper	Ref.		
	1		limit			limit	Value		
	Result:	Since the reference value is outside of the confidence interval, we reject the null hypothesis and accept the research hypothesis.							
	Conclusion:	Respondents to the online survey were significantly dissatisfied with the Elder Care current website.							

Fig. A.8 Answer to Chap. 3: Practice Problem #2

Chapter 3: Practice Problem #3 Answer (see Fig. A.9)

NATIONAL ASSOCIATION OF SOCIAL WORKERS (NASW)

"Find a Job" Site in the Social Work Career Center

Item #16 **"How helpful did you find this site in learning about job possibilities in the field of Social Work?"**

1	2	3	4	5	6	7
Not Helpful						Very Helpful

Rating
5
6
2
3
4
7
5
6
7
7
6
4
5
3
5
6
7
6
5
6
4
3

Null hypothesis: μ = 4

Research hypothesis: μ ≠ 4

n	22
Mean	5.09
STDEV	1.48
s.e.	0.31

95% confidence interval

Lower limit:	4.44
Upper limit:	5.75

Draw a picture of this confidence interval

-----4-----	----4.44----	------------	----5.09----	------------	----5.75----
Ref Value	Lower limit		Mean		Upper Limit

Result: Since the reference value is outside of the confidence interval, we reject the null hypothesis and accept the research hypothesis.

Conclusion: Visitors to the "Find a Job" Web site rated the site in terms of learning about job possibilities in the field of Social Work as significantly helpful.

Fig. A.9 Answer to Chap. 3: Practice Problem #3

Chapter 4: Practice Problem #1 Answer (see Fig. A.10)

MSW SURVEY OF GRADUATES FROM FIVE YEARS AGO

Item #20: **How satisfied are you with the quality of social work education that you received in your MSW program?**

1	2	3	4	5	6	7	8	9
very dissatisfied								very satisfied
		DATA						
		5						
		6		Null hypothesis:		μ	=	5
		4						
		3		Research hypothesis:		μ	≠	5
		7						
		8						
		6		n		19		
		5						
		9		Mean		6.26		
		7						
		6		STDEV		1.69		
		4						
		6		s.e.		0.39		
		8						
		6		critical t		2.101		
		7						
		5		t-test		3.25		
		8						
		9						

Result: Since the absolute value of 3.25 is greater than the critical t of 2.101, we reject the null hypothesis and accept the research hypothesis.

Conclusion: MSW graduates of five years ago were significantly satisfied with the quality of social work education that they received in their MSW program.

Fig. A.10 Answer to Chap. 4: Practice Problem #1

Chapter 4: Practice Problem #2 Answer (see Fig. A.11)

NUMBER OF DAYS FROM REQUEST FOR AN APPOINTMENT TO APPOINTMENT DATE

PATIENT	NO. OF APPOINTMENT DAYS
1	7
2	18
3	12
4	16
5	19
6	21
7	8
8	6
9	4
10	15
11	16
12	18
13	17
14	16
15	12
16	9
17	11
18	14
19	13

Null hypothesis:	μ	=	10 days
Research hypothesis:	μ	≠	10 days

n	19
Mean	13.26
STDEV	4.77
s.e.	1.09
critical t	2.101
t-test	2.98

Result: Since the absolute value of 2.98 is greater than the critical t of 2.101, we reject the null hypothesis and accept the research hypothesis.

Conclusion: The average number of days needed to obtain a primary care appontment was significantly more than 10 days, and was probably closer to 13.3 days.

Fig. A.11 Answer to Chap. 4: Practice Problem #2

Chapter 4: Practice Problem #3 Answer (see Fig. A.12)

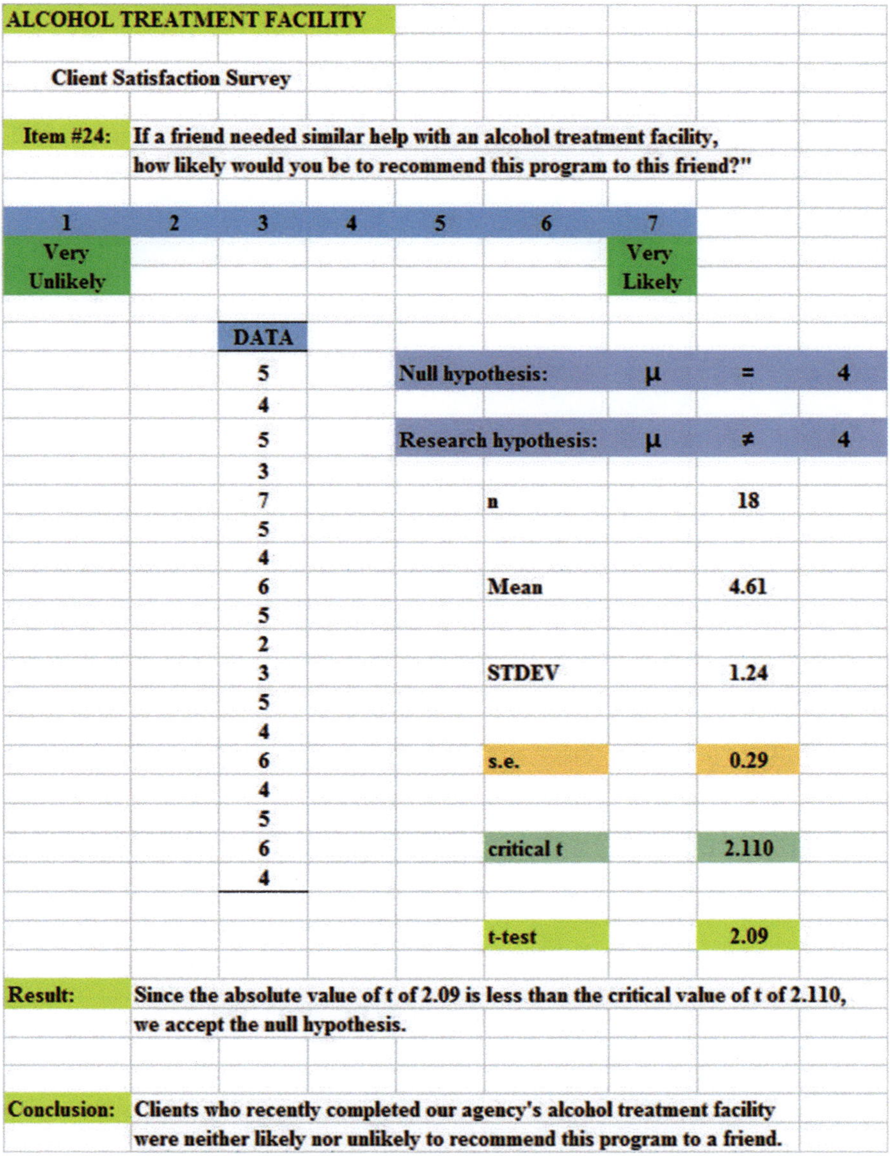

ALCOHOL TREATMENT FACILITY

Client Satisfaction Survey

Item #24: **If a friend needed similar help with an alcohol treatment facility, how likely would you be to recommend this program to this friend?"**

1	2	3	4	5	6	7
Very Unlikely						Very Likely

DATA				
5	Null hypothesis:	μ	=	4
4				
5	Research hypothesis:	μ	≠	4
3				
7		n	18	
5				
4				
6		Mean	4.61	
5				
2				
3		STDEV	1.24	
5				
4				
6		s.e.	0.29	
4				
5				
6		critical t	2.110	
4				
		t-test	2.09	

Result: **Since the absolute value of t of 2.09 is less than the critical value of t of 2.110, we accept the null hypothesis.**

Conclusion: **Clients who recently completed our agency's alcohol treatment facility were neither likely nor unlikely to recommend this program to a friend.**

Fig. A.12 Answer to Chap. 4: Practice Problem #3

Chapter 5: Practice Problem #1 Answer (see Fig. A.13)

BACHELOR OF SOCIAL WORK (BSW) PROGRAM

SENIOR SURVEY

Item #25: **"Overall, how would you rate the quality of the required core courses in the BSW program?**

1	2	3	4	5	6	7	8	9	10
Poor									Excellent

Males	Females
5	6
6	7
4	5
3	8
4	4
6	9
7	6
9	7
5	5
4	6
3	7
2	9
6	
5	

Null hypothesis: $\mu_1 = \mu_2$

Research hypothesis: $\mu_1 \neq \mu_2$

Group	n	Mean	STDEV
1 Males	14	4.93	1.82
2 Females	12	6.58	1.56

(n1 -1) x STDEV1 squared	42.93
(n2 - 1) x STDEV2 squared	26.92
n1 + n2 – 2	24
1/n1 + 1/n2	0.15
s.e.	0.67
critical t (df = n1 + n2 – 2)	2.064
t-test	-2.47

Result: **Since the absolute value of − 2.47 is greater than the critical t of 2.064, we reject the null hypothesis and accept the research hypothesis.**

Conclusion: **Female majors reated the overall quality of the required core courses in the BSW program significantly more positively than male majors in the BSW program (6.58 vs. 4.93).**

Fig. A.13 Answer to Chap. 5: Practice Problem #1

Chapter 5: Practice Problem #2 Answer (see Fig. A.14)

ALCOHOL TREATMENT PROGRAM OUTCOME MEASURE

OVERALL PROGRAM EFFECTIVENESS RATING

Item #15: **"Overall, how would you rate the effectiveness of this alcohol treatment program?**

1	2	3	4	5	6	7
low						high

	MALES	FEMALES
	5	5
	6	4
	7	3
	4	6
ALCOHOL16	3	7
	6	5
	5	6
	8	4
	4	8
	5	5
	6	4
	4	
	5	

Null hypothesis:	μ_1	=	μ_2
Research hypothesis:	μ_1	≠	μ_2

Group	n	Mean	STDEV
1 Males	13	5.23	1.36
2 Females	11	5.18	1.47

(n1 − 1) x STDEV1 squared	22.31
(n2 − 1) x STDEV2 squared	21.64
n1 + n2 − 2	22
1/n1 + 1/n2	0.17
s.e.	0.58
critical t	2.074
t-test	0.08

Result: Since the absolute value of t of 0.08 is less than the critical value of 2.074, we accept the null hypothesis.

Conclusion: There was no difference in the ratings of the effectiveness of the alcohol treatment program beweeen males and females.

Fig. A.14 Answer to Chap. 5: Practice Problem #2

Chapter 5: Practice Problem #3 Answer (see Fig. A.15)

MASTER'S OF SOCIAL WORK (MSW) PROGRAM				
GPA of students who have completed all required core courses				
	H_0 :	μ_1	=	μ_2
	H_1 :	μ_1	≠	μ_2
	Group	n	Mean	STDEV
	1 Males	47	3.15	0.42
MSW12	2 Females	56	3.45	0.37
	STDEV1 squared / n1			0.004
	STDEV2 squared / n2			0.002
	E12 + E14			0.006
	s.e.			0.079
	critical t			1.96
	t-test			− 3.811
Result:	Since the abvolute value of − 3.811 is greater than the critical t of 1.96, we reject the null hypothesis and accept the research hypothesis.			
Conclusion:	Female students in the MSW program had a significantly higher GPA after completing all the required core courses in the program than Male students (3.45 vs. 3.15)			

Fig. A.15 Answer to Chap. 5: Practice Problem #3

Chapter 6: Practice Problem #1 Answer (see Fig. A.16)

EXTENDED FAMILY VISITS vs. DEPRESSION SCORE OF A NURSING HOME RESIDENT

Is there a relationship between the number of visits to the nursing home by extended family members in a month and the depression score of the nursing home resident at the end of that month?

FAMILY VISITS	DEPRESSION SCORE
0	18
2	42
4	52
3	45
5	35
7	41
6	40
8	23
9	15
10	10
correlation	-0.45

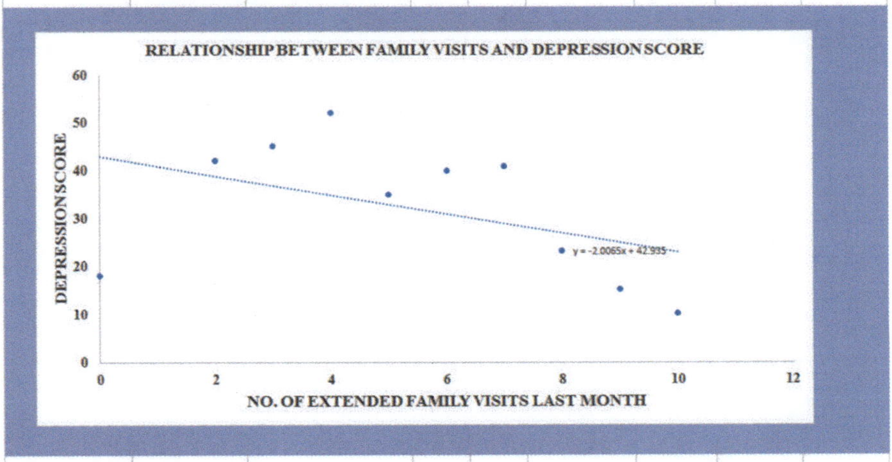

SUMMARY OUTPUT

Regression Statistics	
Multiple R	0.45
R Square	0.199
Adjusted R Square	0.098
Standard Error	13.697
Observations	10

ANOVA

	df	*SS*	*MS*	*F*	*Significance F*
Regression	1	372.004	372.004	1.983	0.197
Residual	8	1500.896	187.612		
Total	9	1872.900			

	Coefficients	*Standard Error*	*t Stat*	*P-value*	*Lower 95%*	*Upper 95%*	*Lower 95.0%*	*Upper 95.0%*
Intercept	42.94	8.830	4.862	0.001	22.573	63.297	22.573	63.297
X Variable 1	-2.01	1.425	-1.408	0.197	-5.292	1.279	-5.292	1.279

Fig. A.16 Answer to Chap. 6: Practice Problem #1

Chapter 6: Practice Problem #1 (continued)

1. $r = -.45$ (Note the negative correlation!)
2. $a = y$ - intercept $= +42.94$
3. $b = \text{slope} = -2.01$ (Note the negative slope!)
4. $Y = a + bX$
   $Y = 42.94 - 2.01X$
5. $Y = 42.94 - 2.01(5)$
   $Y = 42.94 - 10.05$
   $Y = 32.89 = 33$ (as the predicted depression score)

Important note: Look at your final spreadsheet: FAMILY3. If you used the =correl function to find the correlation below the data table, it should be: −.45 (a negative correlation!). Note that the SUMMARY OUTPUT gives a correlation of +.45 because the correlation in this output table will NEVER be a negative correlation because of a huge mistake that the computer programmer made in creating the formula for the correlation (and which the programmer also labeled incorrectly as: "Multiple R", when it should have been labeled: "correlation r" instead.

Chapter 6: Practice Problem #2 Answer (see Fig. A.17)

CASELOAD SIZE vs. NO. OF SICK DAYS IN JULY-DECEMBER OF LAST YEAR

Is there a relationship between the caseload size of workers and the number of sick days they took in the last six months of last year?

CASELOAD	NO. OF SICK DAYS
52	8
55	8
43	8
44	6
49	6
52	5
46	7
46	6
47	7
51	4
54	9
55	10
48	7
49	6
48	7
51	9
56	8
53	11

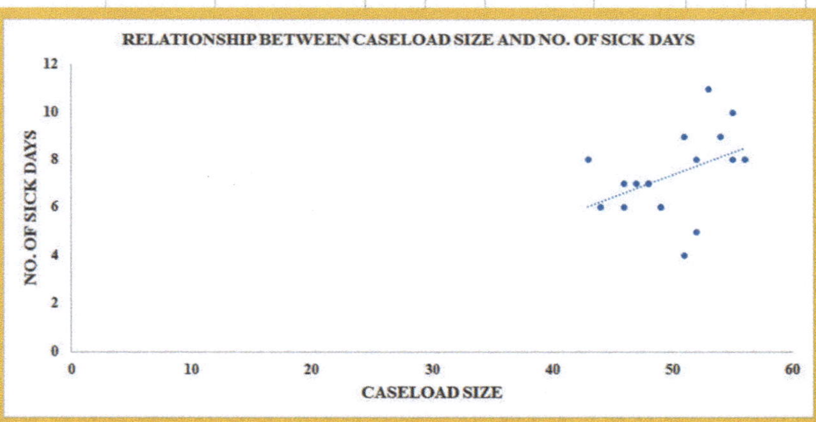

SUMMARY OUTPUT

Regression Statistics	
Multiple R	0.42
R Square	0.1748
Adjusted R Square	0.1233
Standard Error	1.6376
Observations	18

ANOVA

	df	*SS*	*MS*	*F*	*Significance F*
Regression	1	9.0919	9.0919	3.3903	0.0842
Residual	16	42.9081	2.6818		
Total	17	52			

	Coefficients	*Standard Error*	*t Stat*	*P-value*	*Lower 95%*	*Upper 95%*
Intercept	-2.06	5.1170	-0.4029	0.6924	-12.9092	8.7860
X Variable 1	0.19	0.1022	1.8413	0.0842	-0.0285	0.4047

Fig. A.17 Answer to Chap. 6: Practice Problem #2

Chapter 6: Practice Problem #2 (continued)

(2b) about 8 sick days

1. $r = +.42$
2. $a = y\text{-intercept} = -2.06$
3. $b = \text{slope} = +0.19$
4. $Y = a + bX$
   $Y = -2.06 + 0.19X$
5. $Y = -2.06 + 0.19\ (50)$
   $Y = -2.06 + 9.50$
   $Y = 7.44 =$ About 7.5 days

Chapter 6: Practice Problem #3 Answer (see Fig. A.18)

RELATIONSHIP BETWEEN DIET AND WEIGHT LOSS

ADULT WOMEN AGES 30-40

DIET (calories allowed per day)	WEIGHT LOSS (kg)
900	16.0
1050	12.0
1150	8.0
1275	6.0
1420	3.0
1530	5.5
1610	9.5
1710	2.5
1820	6.0
1875	9.0
1930	6.0
2100	3.0

correlation	-0.64

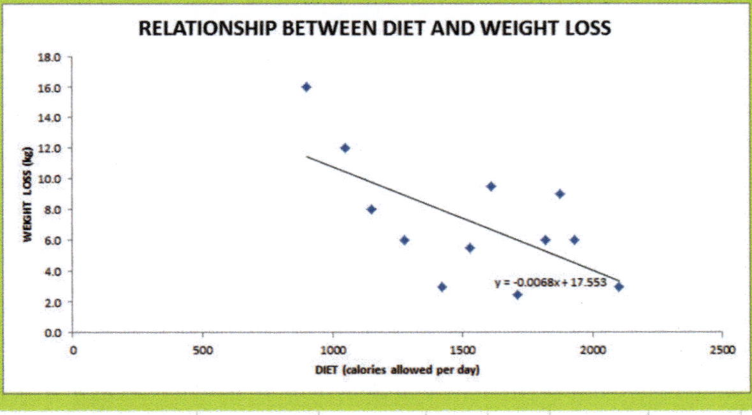

SUMMARY OUTPUT

Regression Statistics	
Multiple R	0.64
R Square	0.413
Adjusted R Square	0.354
Standard Error	3.198
Observations	12

ANOVA

	df	*SS*	*MS*	*F*	*Significance F*
Regression	1	71.946	71.946	7.034	0.024
Residual	10	102.284	10.228		
Total	11	174.229			

	Coefficients	*Standard Error*	*t Stat*	*P-value*	*Lower 95%*	*Upper 95%*
Intercept	17.553	4.008	4.379	0.001	8.622	26.483
X Variable 1	-0.007	0.003	-2.652	0.024	-0.012	-0.001

Fig. A.18 Answer to Chap. 6: Practice Problem #3

Chapter 6: Practice Problem #3 (continued)

1. r = −.64 (Note the negative correlation!)
2. a = y - intercept = 17.553
3. b = slope = − 0.007
4. Y = a + bX
   Y = 17.553 − 0.007X
5. Y = 17.553 − 0.007 (1500)
   Y = 17.553 − 10.5
   Y = 7.053 = 7.1 kg

Chapter 7: Practice Problem #1 Answer (see Fig. A.19)

INSURED POPULATION

RELATIONSHIP BETWEEN VISITS, AGE, AND DISTANCE TO THE NEAREST CLINIC

VISITS	AGE	DISTANCE
5	40	0.3
1	23	7.2
1	18	4.3
7	53	1.5
2	28	6.1
5	25	3.2
5	58	0.2
6	40	2.3
1	25	6.1
8	54	1.3
6	51	1.1
1	20	5.8
3	35	1.4
2	23	5.3
5	51	1.4
5	58	1.1
3	30	2.4

SUMMARY OUTPUT

Regression Statistics	
Multiple R	0.86
R Square	0.741
Adjusted R Square	0.704
Standard Error	1.244
Observations	17

ANOVA

	df	*SS*	*MS*	*F*	*Significance F*
Regression	2	62.098	31.049	20.063	7.74602E-05
Residual	14	21.666	1.548		
Total	16	83.765			

	Coefficients	*Standard Error*	*t Stat*	*P-value*	*Lower 95%*	*Upper 95%*
Intercept	1.8785	2.043	0.920	0.373	-2.503	6.260
AGE	0.0839	0.038	2.224	0.043	0.003	0.165
DISTANCE	-0.3718	0.235	-1.583	0.136	-0.876	0.132

	VISITS	*AGE*	*DISTANCE*
VISITS	1		
AGE	0.83	1	
DISTANCE	-0.81	-0.82	1

Fig. A.19 Answer to Chap. 7: Practice Problem #1

Chapter 7: Practice Problem #1 (continued)

Let X_1 = AGE, and X_2 = DISTANCE

1. Multiple correlation = .86
2. y - intercept = 1.8785
3. $b_1 = 0.0839$
4. $b_2 = -0.3718$
5. $Y = a + b_1X_1 + b_2X_2$
   $Y = 1.8785 + 0.0839\ X_1 - 0.3718\ X_2$
6. $Y = 1.8785 + 0.0839\ (34) - 0.3718\ (5)$
   $Y = 1.8785 + 2.8526 - 1.859$
   $Y = 2.8721$
   Y = almost 3 visits
7. 0.83
8. –0.81
9. –0.82
10. The better predictor of VISITS was AGE ($r = .83$).
11. The two predictors combined predict VISITS at $R_{xy} = .86$, and this is slightly better than the better single predictor by itself.

Chapter 7: Practice Problem #2 Answer (see Fig. A.20)

FINAL EXAM RESULTS IN THE REQUIRED STATISTICS COURSE IN THE BSW PROGRAM

How well do Age, Undergraduate GPA, and SAT Math scores predict Final Exam scores in Statistics?

FINAL EXAM	AGE	GPA	SAT MATH
92	20	3.62	740
88	19	3.45	720
91	21	3.84	680
85	22	2.85	650
75	24	2.50	610
86	21	3.42	620
84	20	3.15	550
85	19	3.64	580
79	25	3.05	590
73	23	2.95	610
76	24	2.84	630
80	22	3.06	620
79	23	3.10	560

SUMMARY OUTPUT

Regression Statistics	
Multiple R	0.90
R Square	0.810
Adjusted R Squa	0.747
Standard Error	3.045
Observations	13

ANOVA

	df	*SS*	*MS*	*F*	*Significance F*
Regression	3	355.772	118.591	12.788	0.001
Residual	9	83.459	9.273		
Total	12	439.231			

	Coefficients	*Standard Error*	*t Stat*	*P-value*	*Lower 95%*	*Upper 95%*
Intercept	59.724	25.311	2.360	0.043	2.466	116.982
AGE	-0.957	0.663	-1.443	0.183	-2.458	0.543
GPA	7.599	3.495	2.174	0.058	-0.307	15.504
SAT MATH	0.031	0.017	1.836	0.100	-0.007	0.069

	FINAL EXAM	AGE	GPA	SAT MATH
FINAL EXAM	1			
AGE	-0.77	1		
GPA	0.83	-0.74	1	
SAT MATH	0.60	-0.35	0.41	1

Fig. A.20 Answer to Chap. 7: Practice Problem #2

Chapter 7: Practice Problem #2 (continued)

Let X_1 = AGE, X_2 = GPA, and X_3 = SAT MATH

1. $R_{xy} = .90$
2. a = y - intercept = 59.724
3. $b_1 = -0.957$
4. $b_2 = 7.599$
5. $b_3 = 0.031$
6. $Y = a + b_1X_1 + b_2X_2 + b_3X_3$
   $Y = 59.724 - 0.957\ X_1 + 7.599\ X_2 + 0.031\ X_3$
7. $Y = 59.724 - 0.957\ (21) + 7.599\ (3.25) + 0.031\ (650)$
   $Y = 59.724 - 20.097 + 24.697 + 20.15$
   $Y = 104.571 - 20.097 = 84.474$ = About 85 on the final exam
8. −0.77
9. 0.83
10. 0.60
11. −0.74
12. 0.41
13. GPA is the best predictor of the final exam score ($r = 0.83$)
14. The three predictors combined predict the final exam score much better than the best single predictor by itself ($R_{xy} = 0.90$)

Chapter 7: Practice Problem #3 Answer (see Fig. A.21)

INSURED POPULATION

VISITS	INCOME ($000)*	DISTANCE (nearest mile)
3	16	8
2	13	10
1	14	12
4	9	2
1	6	12
2	10	11
4	24	3
2	9	12
2	16	10
6	32	4
5	39	3
6	38	2
3	9	5
4	26	5
5	34	2

* INCOME = DISPOSABLE FAMILY INCOME DIVIDED BY FAMILY SIZE

SUMMARY OUTPUT

Regression Statistics	
Multiple R	0.95
R Square	0.912
Adjusted R Square	0.897
Standard Error	0.537
Observations	15

ANOVA

	df	*SS*	*MS*	*F*
Regression	2	35.867	17.934	62.086
Residual	12	3.466	0.289	
Total	14	39.333		

	Coefficients	*Standard Error*	*t Stat*	*P-value*
Intercept	3.818	0.633	6.027	0.000
INCOME ($000)*	0.062	0.017	3.541	0.004
DISTANCE (nearest mile)	-0.252	0.049	-5.137	0.000

	VISITS	INCOME ($000)*	DISTANCE (nearest mile)
VISITS	1		
INCOME ($000)*	0.85	1	
DISTANCE (nearest mile)	-0.91	-0.69	1

Fig. A.21 Answer to Chap. 7: Practice Problem #3

Chapter 7: Practice Problem #3 (continued)

Let X_1 = INCOME, and X_2 = DISTANCE

1. Multiple correlation = .95
2. a = y - intercept = 3.818
3. $b_1 = 0.062$
4. $b_2 = -0.252$
5. $Y = a + b_1X_1 + b_2X_2$
   $Y = 3.818 + 0.062\ X_1 - 0.252\ X_2$
6. $Y = 3.818 + 0.062\ (26) - 0.252\ (4)$
   $Y = 3.818 + 1.612 - 1.008$
   $Y = 4.422$
   Y = 4.4 VISITS
7. +0.85
8. –0.91
9. –0.69
10. The better single predictor of VISITS was DISTANCE (r = –.91).
11. The two predictors combined predicted VISITS slightly better at $R_{xy} = .95$.

Chapter 8: Practice Problem #1 Answer (see Fig. A.22)

	SOURCE OF SOCIAL WORK TEACHING APPLICATIONS					
	NUMBER OF APPLICATIONS					
	CHRONICLE	NASW	CSWE			
	85	68	86			
	64	64	89			
	92	65	102			
	54	62	116			
	68	63	101			
	67	61	98			
	55	60	95			
	82	59	94			
Anova: Single Factor						
SUMMARY						
Groups	*Count*	*Sum*	*Average*	*Variance*		
CHRONICLE	8	567	70.88	196.70		
NASW	8	502	62.75	8.50		
CSWE	8	781	97.63	85.41		
ANOVA						
Source of Variation	*SS*	*df*	*MS*	*F*	*P-value*	*F crit*
Between Groups	5327.58	2.00	2663.79	27.50	0.00	3.47
Within Groups	2034.25	21.00	96.87			
Total	7361.83	23.00				
NASW vs. CSWE						
1/n NASW + 1/n CSWE	0.25					
s.e. NASW vs. CSWE	4.92					
ANOVA t-test	-7.09					

Fig. A.22 Answer to Chap. 8: Practice Problem #1

Chapter 8: Practice Problem #1 (continued)

Let Group 1 = CHRONICLE, Group 2 = NASW, and Group 3 = CSWE

1. $H_0 : \mu_1 = \mu_2 = \mu_3$
   $H_1 : \mu_1 \neq \mu_2 \neq \mu_3$
2. $MS_b = 2663.79$
3. $MSw = 96.87$
4. $F = 2663.79/96.87 = 27.50$
5. critical $F = 3.47$
6. Result: Since 27.50 is greater than 3.47, we reject the null hypothesis and accept the research hypothesis
7. Conclusion: There was a significant difference between the three Web sites in job applications received for a social work teaching position.

   NASW versus CSWE

8. $H_0 : \mu_2 = \mu_3$
   $H_1 : \mu_2 \neq \mu_3$
9. 62.75
10. 97.63
11. $df = n_{TOTAL} - k = 24 - 3 = 21$
12. critical $t = 2.080$
13. $1/8 + 1/8 = 0.125 + 0.125 = 0.25$
    s.e. = SQRT(96.87*0.25) = SQRT(24.22) = 4.92
14. ANOVA $t = (62.75 - 97.63)/4.92 = -34.88/4.92 = -7.09$
15. Result: Since the absolute value of −7.09 is greater than the critical t of 2.080, we reject the null hypothesis and accept the research hypothesis
16. Conclusion: CSWE had significantly more job applications for a social work position than NASW (98 vs. 63).

Chapter 8: Practice Problem #2 Answer (see Fig. A.23)

NUMBER OF DAYS UNTIL TRANSFER TO A NURSING HOME

	HOSPITAL		
A	B	C	D
9	5	15	12
11	9	18	14
12	8	16	16
10	7	17	18
12	6	19	17
11	5	21	13
13	7	22	17
9	9	19	16
14	10		15
10			14
13			

Anova: Single Factor

SUMMARY

Groups	*Count*	*Sum*	*Average*	*Variance*
A	11	124	11.27	2.82
B	9	66	7.33	3.25
C	8	147	18.38	5.70
D	10	152	15.20	3.73

ANOVA

Source of Variation	*SS*	*df*	*MS*	*F*	*P-value*	*F crit*
Between Groups	600.69	3	200.23	53.33	0.00	2.88
Within Groups	127.66	34	3.75			
Total	728.34	37				

HOSPITAL B vs. HOSPITAL C	
1/9+1/8	0.24
s.e. ANOVA	0.94
ANOVA t-test	-11.73

Fig. A.23 Answer to Chap. 8: Practice Problem #2

Chapter 8: Practice Problem #2 (continued)

1. Null hypothesis: $\mu_A = \mu_B = \mu_C = \mu_D$
   Research hypothesis: $\mu_A \neq \mu_B \neq \mu_C \neq \mu_D$
2. $MS_b = 200.23$
3. $MS_w = 3.75$
4. $F = 200.23/3.75 = 53.39$
5. critical $F = 2.88$
6. Since the F-value of 53.39 is greater than the critical F value of 2.88, we reject the null hypothesis and accept the research hypothesis.
7. There was a significant difference between the four hospitals in the number of days to transfer patients to a nursing home.
   HOSPITAL B vs. HOSPITAL C
8. Null hypothesis: $\mu_B = \mu_C$
   Research hypothesis: $\mu_B \neq \mu_C$
9. 7.33
10. 18.38
11. $df = 38 - 4 = 34$
12. critical $t = 2.032$
13. $1/9 + 1/8 = 0.11 + 0.125 = 0.235$
    s.e. = SQRT $(3.75^*0.235)$ = SQRT $(0.8812) = 0.94$
14. ANOVA $t = (7.33 - 18.38)/0.94 = -11.76$
15. Since the absolute value of -11.76 is greater than the critical t of 2.032, we reject the null hypothesis and accept the research hypothesis
16. HOSPITAL C took significantly more days to transfer patients to a nursing home than HOSPITAL B (18.38 VS. 7.33 days)

Chapter 8: Practice Problem #3 Answer (see Fig. A.24)

LENGTH OF STAY (LOS)					
		HEALTH CARE FACILITY			
	A	B	C	D	E
	3	2	3	7	5
	4	8	5	11	9
	5	4	9	12	6
	4	6	6	9	8
	5	7	7	8	7
	3	3	8	6	6
	2	5	4	7	5
	4	8	11	10	9
	5	9	12	12	7
	4	7	10		4
	3		11		6
			9		8
					9

Anova: Single Factor

SUMMARY

Groups	*Count*	*Sum*	*Average*	*Variance*
A	11	42	3.82	0.96
B	10	59	5.90	5.43
C	12	95	7.92	8.63
D	9	82	9.11	5.11
E	13	89	6.85	2.81

ANOVA

Source of Variation	*SS*	*df*	*MS*	*F*	*P-value*	*F crit*
Between Groups	168.07	4	42.02	9.21	0.00	2.56
Within Groups	228.03	50	4.56			
Total	396.11	54				

HOSPITAL B vs. HOSPITAL E	
1/10+1/13	0.18
s.e. ANOVA	0.90
ANOVA t-test	-1.05

Fig. A.24 Answer to Chap. 8: Practice Problem #3

Chapter 8: Practice Problem #3 (continued)

1. Null hypothesis: $\mu_A = \mu_B = \mu_C = \mu_D = \mu_E$
   Research hypothesis: $\mu_A \neq \mu_B \neq \mu_C \neq \mu_D \neq \mu_E$
2. $MS_b = 42.02$
3. $MS_w = 4.56$
4. F = 42.02/4.56 = 9.21
5. critical F = 2.56
6. Result: Since the F-value of 9.21 is greater than the critical F value of 2.56, we reject the null hypothesis and accept the research hypothesis.
7. Conclusion: There was a significant difference between the five types of health care facilities in their length of stay of inpatients.

   HEALTH CARE FACILITY B vs. HEALTH CARE FACILITY E

8. Null hypothesis: $\mu_B = \mu_E$
   Research hypothesis: $\mu_B \neq \mu_E$
9. 5.90
10. 6.85
11. degrees of freedom = 55 − 5 = 50
12. critical t = 1.96
13. $\text{s.e.}_{\text{ANOVA}} = \text{SQRT}(MS_w \times \{1/10 + 1/13\})$
    $= \text{SQRT}\ (4.56 \times 0.18)$
    $= \text{SQRT}\ (0.82) = 0.91$
14. ANOVA t = (5.90 − 6.85)/0.91 = − 1.04
15. Since the absolute value of −1.04 is less than the critical t of 1.96, we accept the null hypothesis.
16. There was no difference between HEALTH CARE FACILITY B and HEALTH CARE FACILITY E in length of stay (LOS).

Appendix B: Practice Test

Chapter 1: Practice Test

The Master of Social Work program (MSW) at the University of Missouri-St. Louis in St. Louis, Missouri USA is accredited by the Council on Social Work Education. A course in statistics is one of the required courses in this program. Suppose that you have asked to create a table that summarizes the final exam performance of students (100 points possible) in this course during the past semester. You want to try out your Excel skills on a small sample of students, and you have created the hypothetical data given in Fig. B.1.

UNIVERSITY OF MISSOURI- ST. LOUIS MSW PROGRAM

FINAL EXAM SCORES FOR STATISTICS

SCORE
85
92
91
85
83
75
76
81
92
78
84
71
65
72

Fig. B.1 Worksheet Data for Chap. 1 Practice Test (Practical Example)

(a) Create an Excel table for these data, and then use Excel to the right of the table to find the sample size, mean, standard deviation, and standard error of the mean for these data. Label your answers, and round off the mean, standard deviation, and standard error of the mean to two decimal places.
(b) Save the file as: FINAL3

Chapter 2: Practice Test

A health care facility has discharged 124 patients within the last 60 days. Suppose that you want to do a Customer Satisfaction Survey on a random sample of 20 of these 124 patients for this survey.

(a) Set up a spreadsheet of frame numbers for these patients with the heading: FRAME NUMBERS
(b) Then, create a separate column to the right of these frame numbers which duplicates these frame numbers with the title: Duplicate frame numbers.
(c) Then, create a separate column to the right of these duplicate frame numbers called RAND NO. and use the *=RAND()* function to assign random numbers to all of the frame numbers in the duplicate frame numbers column. Change this column format so that three decimal places appear for each random number.
(d) Sort the *duplicate frame numbers and random numbers* into a random order.
(e) Print the result so that the spreadsheet fits onto one page.
(f) Circle on your printout the I.D. number of the first 20 patients that you would use in your survey.
(g) Save the file as: RAND58

Important note: Everyone who does this problem will generate a different random order of patient ID numbers since Excel assigns a different random number each time the RAND() command is used. For this reason, the answer to this problem given in this Excel Guide will have a completely different sequence of random numbers from the random sequence that you generate. This is normal and is to be expected.

Chapter 3: Practice Test

The Master of Social Work (MSW) program at the Brown School of Social Work at Washington University in St. Louis, Missouri USA is fully accredited by the Council of Social Work Education. One of the concentrations in this MSW program is in "Older Adults and Aging Societies." Suppose that you have been asked to do the data analysis for a Survey of graduate students in this concentration two months before they were scheduled to complete their MSW degree. The survey is intended to obtain feedback from these students about the quality of their MSW program. The survey is in its early stages of development, but you have been told that Item #25 of this survey will ask the students to rate the overall quality of the MSW program on a 9-point rating scale. You want to test your Excel skills, so you have developed some hypothetical data for this item that are given in Fig. B.2.

WASHINGTON UNIVERSITY IN ST. LOUIS, MISSOURI								
THE BROWN SCHOOL MASTER OF SOCIAL WORK PROGRAM								
ITEM #25:	"Overall, how would you rate the quality of the MSW program							
	at Washington University in St. Louis?"							
1	2	3	4	5	6	7	8	9
Poor								Excellent
	RATING							
	6							
	8							
	5							
	4							
	6							
	7							
	5							
	3							
	6							
	2							
	4							
	9							
	7							
	6							
	8							
	7							
	8							
	9							

Fig. B.2 Worksheet Data for Chap. 3 Practice Test (Practical Example)

(a) Create an Excel table for these data, and use Excel to the right of the table to find the sample size, mean, standard deviation, and standard error of the mean for these data. Label your answers, and round off the mean, standard deviation, and standard error of the mean to two decimal places in number format.
(b) By hand, write the null hypothesis and the research hypothesis on your printout.
(c) Use Excel's *TINV function* to find the 95% confidence interval about the mean for these data. Label your answers. Use two decimal places for the confidence interval figures in number format.
(d) On your printout, draw a diagram of this 95% confidence interval by hand, including the reference value.
(e) On your spreadsheet, enter the *result.*
(f) On your spreadsheet, enter the *conclusion in plain English.*
(g) Print the data and the results so that your spreadsheet fits onto one page.
(h) Save the file as: MSW26

Chapter 4: Practice Test

The American College of Healthcare Executives (ACHE) is an international professional association that has more than 40,000 healthcare executives as members. ACHE holds an annual Congress on Healthcare Leadership which draws more than 4,500 participants from around the world to Chicago, Illinois (USA). ACHE offers a variety of educational programs. One format that it is using allows members to attend online Webinars, instead of having to spend travel funds and time to go to seminars in cities around the world. Suppose that you have been asked to develop a survey that can be emailed to members who have taken a Webinar to determine their preference for that method of presentation. You are sure that you want to include an item that deals with the extent to which Webinar participants prefer that method of educational delivery, and you want to test your Excel skills on a small sample of data using the hypothetical data given in Fig. B.3.

AMERICAN COLLEGE OF HEALTHCARE EXECUTIVES (ACHE)						
Survey of Educational Programs						
ITEM #10:	How much do you prefer or not prefer to have the educational programs of ACHE presented in Webinar format?					
1	2	3	4	5	6	7
Do not prefer						Prefer
	RATING					
	2					
	6					
	7					
	5					
	4					
	3					
	6					
	2					
	1					
	5					
	6					
	7					
	3					
	5					
	6					
	4					
	7					
	6					
	5					
	6					
	7					

Fig. B.3 Worksheet Data for Chap. 4 Practice Test (Practical Example)

(a) Write the null hypothesis and the research hypothesis on your spreadsheet.
(b) Create a spreadsheet for these data, and then use Excel to find the sample size, mean, standard deviation, and standard error of the mean to the right of the data set. Use number format (two decimal places) for the mean, standard deviation, and standard error of the mean.
(c) Type the *critical t* from the t-table in Appendix E onto your spreadsheet, and label it.
(d) Use Excel to compute the t-test value for these data (use two decimal places) and label it on your spreadsheet.
(e) Type the *result* on your spreadsheet, and then type the *conclusion in plain English* on your spreadsheet.
(f) Save the file as: RATING10

Chapter 5: Practice Test

The National Association of Social Workers (NASW) includes more than 132,000 social workers in the world as its members. NASW has chapters in all 50 states of the USA. The Web site includes a Professional Education and Training Center (PETC) that specializes as a continuing education resource center for its members. PETC includes an online Webinar continuing education resource that social workers can use 24 hours a day wherever they are located. There are no travel costs involved, obviously, no lost time away from work, and all courses are NASW accredited. Suppose that you have been asked to design an online survey that can be emailed to members of NASW who have completed this Webinar within the past three months: "Anxiety and Social Angst: Approaches to Manage Aging, Chronic Illness, or Disability." You are in the early stages of survey design, but you have decided that you do want to include the rating scale below as Item #20 in this online survey. You want to test your Excel skills on this type of survey, and so you have created the hypothetical data for this one item that are given in Fig. B.4.

NATIONAL ASSOCIATION OF SOCIAL WORKERS (NASW)		
PROFESSIONAL EDUCATION AND TRAINING CENTER (PETC)		
WEBINAR COURSE:	"Anxiety and Social Angst: Approaches to Manage Aging, Chronic Illness, or Disability"	
ITEM #20:	"Overall, how would you rate the value of this Webinar course to your professional development as a social worker?"	

1	2	3	4	5	6	7
Low						High

MALES	FEMALES
6	4
2	5
3	7
5	6
7	5
5	6
6	7
4	5
3	6
1	7
5	4
6	6
7	7
6	6
5	7
7	6
6	7
7	6
5	7
	5
	6
	7

Fig. B.4 Worksheet Data for Chap. 5 Practice Test (Practical Example)

(a) Write the null hypothesis and the research hypothesis.
(b) Create an Excel table that summarizes these data.
(c) Use Excel to find the standard error of the difference of the means.
(d) Use Excel to perform a *two-group t-test*. What is the value of *t* that you obtain (use two decimal places)?
(e) On your spreadsheet, type the *critical value of t* using the t-table in Appendix E.
(f) Type the *result* of the test on your spreadsheet.
(g) Type your *conclusion in plain English* on your spreadsheet.
(h) Save the file as: WEB3
(i) Print the final spreadsheet so that it fits onto one page.

Chapter 6: Practice Test

A healthcare administrator at a large multi-institutional organization (ABC) wants to do a "employee satisfaction survey" with managers at the different locations and has asked you to design a survey that can be sent via email to a random sample of managers. You have not yet completed the design of the survey, but know that you want to include items that ask the managers how satisfied they are with their jobs and also their likelihood their leaving employment at ABC sometime during the next two years. Suppose you want to study this relationship using the hypothetical data for Item 18 and item 30 in your current working draft of the survey and want to test your Excel skills on the hypothetical data that are given in Fig. B.5.

HEALTHCARE FACILITY ABC

EMPLOYEE SATISFACTION SURVEY

Item #18: **"How likely are you to leave employment at ABC sometime in the next two years?"**

1	2	3	4	5	6	7
very unlikely						very likely

Item #30: **"Overall, how satisfied are you with your current job at ABC?"**

1	2	3	4	5	6	7
very dissatisfied						very satisfied

ITEM 30	ITEM 18
2	5
6	6
4	3
3	2
5	4
4	7
3	6
2	5
1	6
4	7
5	4
3	3
6	2
7	1
5	2
4	3
3	1
4	7
2	6
1	6

Fig. B.5 Worksheet Data for Chap. 6 Practice Test (Practical Example)

Create an Excel spreadsheet, and enter the data.

(a) create an *XY scatterplot* of these two sets of data such that:

- top title: RELATIONSHIP BETWEEN JOB SATISFACTION AND LIKELIHOOD OF LEAVING ABC
- x-axis title: JOB SATISFACTION
- y-axis title: LIKELIHOOD OF LEAVING ABC
- move the chart below the table
- re-size the chart so that it is 7 columns wide and 25 rows long
- delete the legend
- delete the gridlines

(b) Create the *least-squares regression line* for these data on the scatterplot.

(c) Use Excel to run the regression statistics to find the *equation for the least-squares regression line* for these data and display the results below the chart on your spreadsheet. Use number format (two decimal places) for the correlation and three decimal places for the coefficients

Print *just the input data and the chart* so that this information fits onto one page in portrait format.

Then, print *just the regression output table* on a separate page so that it fits onto one page.

By hand:

(d) Circle and label the value of the *y-intercept* and the *slope* of the regression line on your printout.

(e) Write the regression equation *by hand* on your printout for these data (use three decimal places for the y-intercept and the slope).

(f) Circle and label the *correlation* between the two sets of scores in the regression analysis summary output table on your printout.

(g) Underneath the regression equation you wrote by hand on your printout, use the regression equation to predict the likelihood of leaving ABC employment for a manager with a job satisfaction score of 3.

(h) Estimate *from the graph*, the average likelihood of leaving ABC you would predict for a manager with a job satisfaction score of 6, and write your answer in the space immediately below:

____

(i) save the file as: SATIS10

Chapter 7: Practice Test

The Graduate Record Examination (GRE) is a standardized test that is an admissions requirement for many U.S. graduate schools that offer an MSW degree. The GRE is intended to measure academic preparedness, regardless of specialization field. Let's suppose that you have been hired as a research assistant by a Director of a Master of Social Work (MSW) program at a major university and that the Director has asked you to find the relationship between GRE VERBAL (score range: 130–170), GRE QUANTITATIVE (score range: 130–170), and GRE WRITING (score range: 0–6) in terms of their ability to predict the first-year GPA for students in this program. In addition, the Director has asked you to add a fourth predictor, UNDERGRADUATE GPA, to your analysis. You want to test your Excel skills, so you have created the hypothetical data in Fig. B.6.

GRADUATE RECORD EXAMINATIONS

How well does the GRE and undergraduate GPA predict a student's GPA at the end of the first year of a Masters' program in Social Work?

FIRST-YEAR GPA	GRE VERBAL	GRE QUANTITATIVE	GRE WRITING	UNDERGRADUATE GPA
3.25	160	161	5	3.40
3.42	156	158	4	3.15
2.85	156	157	2	3.05
2.65	154	153	1	2.55
3.65	166	166	6	3.25
3.16	159	160	3	3.20
3.56	166	163	4	3.66
2.35	155	154	2	2.55
2.86	153	154	3	2.85
2.95	158	157	4	2.80
3.15	158	159	4	3.05
3.45	160	160	5	3.44

Fig. B.6 Worksheet Data for Chap. 7 Practice Test (Practical Example)

(a) create an Excel spreadsheet using FIRST-YEAR GPA as the dependent (criterion) variable (Y), and the other variables as the four predictors of this criterion (X_1 = VERBAL, X_2 = QUANTITATIVE, X_3 = WRITING, and X_4 = UNDERGRADUATE GPA).

(b) Use Excel's *multiple regression* function to find the relationship between these five variables and place the SUMMARY OUTPUT below the table.

(c) Use number format (two decimal places) for the multiple correlation on the Summary Output, and use three decimal places for the coefficients in the SUMMARY OUTPUT.

(d) Save the file as: GRE33

(e) Print the table and regression results below the table so that they fit onto one page.

Answer the following questions using your Excel printout:

1. What is the multiple correlation R_{xy}?
2. What is the y-intercept *a*?
3. What is the coefficient for VERBAL, b_1?
4. What is the coefficient for QUANTITATIVE, b_2?
5. What is the coefficient for WRITING, b_3?

6. What is the coefficient for UNDERGRADUATE GPA, b_4?
7. What is the multiple regression equation?
8. Predict the FIRST-YEAR GPA you would expect for a VERBAL score of 165, a QUANTITATIVE SCORE OF 160, a WRITING SCORE of 4, and an UNDERGRADUATE GPA of 3.10.

(f) Now, go back to your Excel file and create a correlation matrix for these five variables, and place it underneath the SUMMARY OUTPUT.
(g) Re-save this file as: GRE33
(h) Now, print out *just this correlation matrix* on a separate sheet of paper.

Answer the following questions using your Excel printout. (Be sure to include the plus or minus sign for each correlation):

9. What is the correlation between VERBAL and FIRST-YEAR GPA?
10. What is the correlation between QUANTITATIVE and FIRST-YEAR GPA?
11. What is the correlation between WRITING and FIRST-YEAR GPA?
12. What is the correlation between UNDERFGRADUATE GPA and FIRST-YEAR GPA?
13. What is the correlation between VERBAL and QUANTITATIVE?
14. What is the correlation between QUANTITATIVE and WRITING?
15. What is the correlation between WRITING and UNDERGRADUATE GPA?
16. What is the correlation between QUANTITATIVE and UNDERGRADUATE GPA?
17. Discuss which of the four predictors is the best predictor of FIRST-YEAR GPA.
18. Explain in words how much better the four predictor variables combined predict FIRST-YEAR GPA than the best single predictor by itself.

Chapter 8: Practice Test

A budget request from a long-term care facility needs to be based, in part, on the complexity of care required by each resident A healthcare administrator wants to determine the case complexity by comparing a random sample of patients from three facilities (A, B, C) that are part of this multi-institutional organization on the number of secondary diagnoses required by adult women patients (ages 50–60) who have been admitted to the facilities during the twelve months preceding the past 60 days. You decide to test your Excel skills on a small sample of residents from each of three facilities, and you have created the hypothetical data given in Fig. B.7.

CASE COMPLEXITY OF RESIDENTS (Adult women, ages 50-60)			
Number of secondary diagnoses required			
	FACILITY A	FACILITY B	FACILITY C
	2	3	3
	4	5	6
	8	6	4
	6	4	5
	3	7	9
	7	8	7
	2	6	6
	4	1	8
	3	2	6
	5	5	7
	1	3	5
	3	4	6
	4	6	4
	2		5
	5		8
			10

Fig. B.7 Worksheet Data for Chap. 8 Practice Test (Practical Example)

(a) Enter these data on an Excel spreadsheet.

Let FACILITY A = Group 1, FACILITY B = Group 2, and FACILITY C = Group 3.

(b) On your spreadsheet, write the null hypothesis and the research hypothesis for these data.
(c) Perform a *one-way ANOVA test* on these data, and show the resulting ANOVA table underneath the input data for the three facilities.
(d) If the F-value in the ANOVA table is significant, create an Excel formula to compute the ANOVA t-test comparing FACILITY B versus FACILITY C, and show the results below the ANOVA table on the spreadsheet (put the standard error and the ANOVA t-test value on separate lines of your spreadsheet, and use two decimal places for each value)
(e) Print out the resulting spreadsheet so that all of the information fits onto one page
(f) On your printout, label by hand the MS (between groups) and the MS (within groups)
(g) Circle and label the value for F on your printout for the ANOVA of the input data

(h) Label by hand on the printout the mean for FACILITY B and the mean for FACILITY C that were produced by your ANOVA.
(i) Save the spreadsheet as: SECONDARY3

On a separate sheet of paper, now do the following by hand:

(j) Find the critical value of F in the ANOVA Single Factor results table.
(k) Write a summary of the *result* of the ANOVA test for the input data.
(l) Write a summary of the *conclusion* of the ANOVA test in plain English for the input data.
(m) Write the null hypothesis and the research hypothesis comparing FACILITY B versus FACILITY C.
(n) Compute the degrees of freedom for the *ANOVA t-test* by hand for three types of facilities.
(o) Use your calculator and Excel to compute the standard error (s.e.) of the ANOVA t-test.
(p) Use your calculator and Excel to compute the ANOVA t-test value.
(q) Write the *critical value of t* for the ANOVA t-test using the table in Appendix E.
(r) Write a summary of the *result* of the ANOVA t-test.
(s) Write a summary of the *conclusion* of the ANOVA t-test in plain English.

Appendix C: Answers to Practice Test

Practice Test Answer: Chapter 1 (see. Fig. C.1)

UNIVERSITY OF MISSOURI- ST. LOUIS MSW PROGRAM

FINAL EXAM SCORES FOR STATISTICS

SCORE		
85		
92	n	14
91		
85		
83	Mean	80.71
75		
76		
81	STDEV	8.29
92		
78		
84	s.e.	2.21
71		
65		
72		

Fig. C.1 Practice Test Answer to Chap. 1 Problem

Practice Test Answer: Chapter 2 (see. Fig. C.2)

FRAME NUMBERS	Duplicate frame numbers	RAND NO.
1	54	0.879
2	69	0.220
3	34	0.216
4	47	0.788
5	63	0.941
6	16	0.579
7	78	0.587
8	4	0.186
9	113	0.540
10	71	0.114
11	85	0.305
12	91	0.007
13	56	0.155
14	28	0.697
15	1	0.192
16	45	0.649
17	40	0.982
18	108	0.548
19	43	0.545
20	92	0.382
21	61	0.674
22	100	0.577
23		…68
	102	0.…
110	73	0.879
111	81	0.011
112	15	0.590
113	31	0.436
114	2	0.939
115	53	0.119
116	82	0.965
117	5	0.766
118	36	0.026
119	65	0.465
120	58	0.115
121	107	0.190
122	50	0.059
123	11	0.753
124	12	0.245

Fig. C.2 Practice Test Answer to Chap. 2 Problem

Practice Test Answer: Chapter 3 (see. Fig. C.3)

WASHINGTON UNIVERSITY IN ST. LOUIS, MISSOURI

THE BROWN SCHOOL MASTER OF SOCIAL WORK PROGRAM

ITEM #25: "Overall, how would you rate the quality of the MSW program at Washington University in St. Louis?"

1	2	3	4	5	6	7	8	9
Poor								Excellent

RATING
6
8
5
4
6
7
5
3
6
2
4
9
7
6
8
7
8
9

Null hypothesis: μ = 5

Research hypothesis: μ ≠ 5

n	18
Mean	6.11
STDEV	2.00
s.e.	0.47

95% confidence interval

Lower limit: 5.12

Upper limit: 7.10

Draw a picture of the confidence interval

-----5------	------5.12-----	------6.11--	---------7.10-----
Ref Value	Lower Limit	Mean	Upper Limit

Result: Since the reference value is outside of the confidence interval, we reject the null hypothesis and accept the research hypothesis.

Conclusion: Overall, students in the MSW program two months before graduation rated the quality of the MSW program as significantly positive.

Note: ***In the English language, it is not correct th say that something is "significantly excellent" since something is either excellent or not excellent. To avoid this language pitfall, it is much better to refer to a positive opinion as "significantly positive."***

Fig. C.3 Practice Test Answer to Chap. 3 Problem

Practice Test Answer: Chapter 4 (see. Fig. C.4)

AMERICAN COLLEGE OF HEALTHCARE EXECUTIVES (ACHE)							
Survey of Educational Programs							
ITEM #10:	How much do you prefer or not prefer to have the educational programs of ACHE presented in Webinar format?						
1	2	3	4	5	6	7	
Do not prefer						Prefer	
	RATING						
	2		Null hypothesis:		μ	=	4
	6						
	7		Research hypothesis:		μ	≠	4
	5						
	4						
	3			n	21		
	6						
	2						
	1			Mean	4.90		
	5						
	6						
	7			STDEV	1.81		
	3						
	5						
	6			s.e.	0.40		
	4						
	7						
	6			critical t	2.086		
	5						
	6						
	7			t-test	2.29		
		Result:	Since the absolute value of 2.29 is greater than the critical t of 2.086, we reject the null hypothesis and accept the research hypothesis.				
		Conclusion:	Members of ACHE who enrolled in an ACHE Webinar seminar during the past year significantly preferred this type of format for the educational program.				

Fig. C.4 Practice Test Answer to Chap. 4 Problem

Practice Test Answer: Chapter 5 (see. Fig. C.5)

NATIONAL ASSOCIATION OF SOCIAL WORKERS (NASW)

PROFESSIONAL EDUCATION AND TRAINING CENTER (PETC)

WEBINAR COURSE: **"Anxiety and Social Angst: Approaches to Manage Aging, Chronic Illness, or Disability"**

ITEM #20: **"Overall, how would you rate the value of this Webinar course to your professional development as a social worker?"**

1	2	3	4	5	6	7
Low						High

MALES	FEMALES
6	4
2	5
3	7
5	6
7	5
5	6
6	7
4	5
3	6
1	7
5	4
6	6
7	7
6	6
5	7
7	6
6	7
7	6
5	7
	5
	6
	7

$H_0: \mu_1 = \mu_2$

$H_1: \mu_1 \neq \mu_2$

Group	n	Mean	STDEV
1 MALES	19	5.05	1.75
2 FEMALES	22	6.00	0.98

(n1 – 1) x STDEV1 squared	54.95
(n2 – 1) x STDEV2 squared	20.00
n1 + n2 – 2	39
1/n1 + 1/n2	0.10
s.e.	0.43
critical t	2.023
t-test	-2.18

Result: **Since the absolute value of – 2.18 is greater than the critical t of 2.023, we reject the null hypothesis and accept the research hypothesis.**

Conclusion: **Females rated the overall value of this Webinar course to their professional development as a social worker as significantly higher than Males (6.00 vs. 5.05).**

Fig. C.5 Practice Test Answer to Chap. 5 Problem

Practice Test Answer: Chapter 6 (see. Fig. C.6)

HEALTHCARE FACILITY ABC

EMPLOYEE SATISFACTION SURVEY

Item #18: "How likely are you to leave employment at ABC sometime in the next two years?"

1	2	3	4	5	6	7
very unlikely						very likely

Item #30: "Overall, how satisfied are you with your current job at ABC?"

1	2	3	4	5	6	7
very dissatisfied						very satisfied

ITEM 30	ITEM 18
2	5
6	6
4	3
3	2
5	4
4	7
3	6
2	5
1	6
4	7
5	4
3	3
6	2
7	1
5	2
4	3
3	1
4	7
2	6
1	6

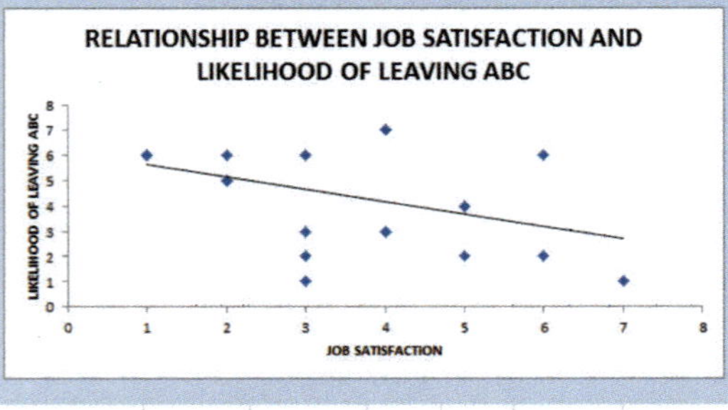

SUMMARY OUTPUT

Regression Statistics	
Multiple R	0.39
R Square	0.1517
Adjusted R Square	0.1046
Standard Error	1.9441
Observations	20

ANOVA

	df	*SS*	*MS*	*F*	*Significance F*
Regression	1	12.1655	12.1655	3.2187	0.0896
Residual	18	68.0345	3.7797		
Total	19	80.2000			

	Coefficients	*Standard Error*	*t Stat*	*P-value*	*Lower 95%*
Intercept	6.086	1.0864	5.6022	0.0000	3.8038
X Variable 1	-0.483	0.2691	-1.7941	0.0896	-1.0481

Fig. C.6 Practice Test Answer to Chap. 6 Problem

Practice Test Answer: Chapter 6: (continued)

(d) a = y-intercept = 6.086

b = slope = -0.483(note the negative sign!)

(e) Y = a + bX

Y = 6.086 – 0.483X

(f) r = correlation = – .39(note the negative sign !)

(g) Y = 6.086 – 0.483(3)

Y = 6.086 – 1.449

Y = 4.637 = 4.6

(h) About 3.3

Practice Test Answer: Chapter 7 (see. Fig. C.7)

GRADUATE RECORD EXAMINATIONS

How well does the GRE and undergraduate GPA predict a student's GPA at the end of the first year of a Masters' program in Social Work?

FIRST-YEAR GPA	GRE VERBAL	GRE QUANTITATIVE	GRE WRITING	UNDERGRAD GPA
3.25	160	161	5	3.40
3.42	156	158	4	3.15
2.85	156	157	2	3.05
2.65	154	153	1	2.55
3.65	166	166	6	3.25
3.16	159	160	3	3.20
3.56	166	163	4	3.66
2.35	155	154	2	2.55
2.86	153	154	3	2.85
2.95	158	157	4	2.80
3.15	158	159	4	3.05
3.45	160	160	5	3.44

SUMMARY OUTPUT

Regression Statistics	
Multiple R	**0.94**
R Square	**0.8825**
Adjusted R Square	**0.8154**
Standard Error	**0.1676**
Observations	**12**

ANOVA

	df	*SS*	*MS*	*F*	*Significance F*
Regression	**4**	**1.4777**	**0.3694**	**13.1467**	**0.0023**
Residual	**7**	**0.1967**	**0.0281**		
Total	**11**	**1.6744**			

	Coefficients	*Standard Error*	*t Stat*	*P-value*	*Lower 95%*
Intercept	**-3.241**	**4.3231**	**-0.7496**	**0.4779**	**-13.4632**
GRE VERBAL	**-0.018**	**0.0388**	**-0.4590**	**0.6601**	**-0.1094**
GRE QUANTITATIVE	**0.046**	**0.0561**	**0.8237**	**0.4373**	**-0.0865**
GRE WRITING	**0.076**	**0.0654**	**1.1589**	**0.2845**	**-0.0789**
UNDERGRADUATE GPA	**0.510**	**0.2642**	**1.9303**	**0.0949**	**-0.1147**

	FIRST-YEAR GPA	*GRE VERBAL*	*GRE QUANTITATIVE*	*GRE WRITING*	*UNDERGRAD GPA*
FIRST-YEAR GPA	**1**				
GRE VERBAL	**0.79**	**1**			
GRE QUANTITATIVE	**0.88**	**0.94**	**1**		
GRE WRITING	**0.83**	**0.72**	**0.83**	**1**	
UNDERGRADUATE GPA	**0.88**	**0.77**	**0.83**	**0.70**	**1**

Fig. C.7 Practice Test Answer to Chap. 7 Problem

Practice Test Answer: Chapter 7 (continued)

1. $R_{xy} = .94$
2. $a = y\text{-intercept} = -3.241$
3. $b_1 = -0.018$
4. $b_2 = 0.046$
5. $b_3 = 0.076$
6. $b_4 = 0.510$
7. $Y = a + b_1X_1 + b_2X_2 + b_3X_3 + b_4X_4$
   $Y = -3.241 - 0.018\ X_1 + 0.046\ X_2 + 0.076\ X_3 + 0.510\ X_4$
8. $Y = -3.241 - 0.018\ (165) + 0.046\ (160) + 0.076\ (4) + 0.510\ (3.10)$
   $Y = -3.241 - 2.97 + 7.36 + 0.30 + 1.58$
   $Y = 9.24 - 6.21 = 3.03$ GPA
9. +.79
10. +.88
11. +.83
12. +.88
13. +.94
14. +.83
15. +.70
16. +.83
17. The best predictor of FIRST-YEAR GPA was a tie between UNDERGRADUATE GPA and QUANTITATIVE since both had a correlation of +.88 with FIRST-YEAR GPA.
18. The four predictors combined predict FIRST-YEAR GPA much better ($R_{xy} = .94$) than the two best single predictors by themselves.

Practice Test Answer: Chapter 8 (see. Fig. C.8)

CASE COMPLEXITY OF RESIDENTS (Adult women, ages 50-60)

$H_0: \mu_1 = \mu_2 = \mu_3$

$H_1: \mu_1 \neq \mu_2 \neq \mu_3$

Number of secondary diagnoses required

FACILITY A	FACILITY B	FACILITY C
2	3	3
4	5	6
8	6	4
6	4	5
3	7	9
7	8	7
2	6	6
4	1	8
3	2	6
5	5	7
1	3	5
3	4	6
4	6	4
2		5
5		8
		10

Anova: Single Factor

SUMMARY

Groups	*Count*	*Sum*	*Average*	*Variance*
FACILITY A	15	59	3.93	3.92
FACILITY B	13	60	4.62	4.09
FACILITY C	16	99	6.19	3.63

ANOVA

Source of Variation	*SS*	*df*	*MS*	*F*	*P-value*	*F crit*
Between Groups	41.46	2	20.73	5.36	0.01	3.23
Within Groups	158.45	41	3.86			
Total	199.91	43				

FACILITY B vs. FACILITY C

1/n FACILITY B + 1/n FACILITY C	0.14
s.e. FACILITY B vs. FACILITY C	0.73
ANOVA t-test	-2.14

Fig. C.8 Practice Test Answer to Chap. 8 Problem

Practice Test Answer: Chapter 8 (continued)

Let FACILITY A = Group 1, FACILITY B = Group 2, and FACILITY C = Group 3.

(b) $H_0: \mu_1 = \mu_2 = \mu_3$
$H_1: \mu_1 \neq \mu_2 \neq \mu_3$

(f) $MS_b = 20.73$ and $MS_w = 3.86$

(g) F = 5.36

(h) Mean of FACILITY B = 4.62 and Mean of FACILITY C = 6.19

(j) critical F = 3.23

(k) Result: Since 5.36 is greater than 3.23, we reject the null hypothesis and accept the research hypothesis

(l) Conclusion: There was a significant difference in required secondary diagnoses for adult women aged 50-60 between the three facilities.

(m) $H_0: \mu_2 = \mu_3$
$H_1: \mu_2 \neq \mu_3$

(n) $df = n_{TOTAL} - k = 44 - 3 = 41$

(o) $1/13 + 1/16 = 0.077 + 0.063 = 0.14$
s.e = SQRT (3.86* 0.14)
s.e. = SQRT (0.54)
s.e. = 0.74

(p) ANOVA t = (4.62 – 6.19)/0.74 = – 2.12 (note the negative sign !)

(q) critical t = 1.96

(r) Result: Since the absolute value of –2.12 is greater than the critical t of 1.96, we reject the null hypothesis and accept the research hypothesis.

(s) Conclusion: FACILITY C had significantly more required secondary diagnoses than FACILITY B (6.19 vs. 4.62).

Appendix D: Statistical Formulas

Mean $$\bar{X} = \frac{\sum X}{n}$$

Standard Deviation $$\text{STDEV} = S = \sqrt{\frac{\sum (X - \bar{X})^2}{n - 1}}$$

Standard error of the mean $$\text{s.e.} = S_{\bar{X}} = \frac{S}{\sqrt{n}}$$

Confidence interval about the mean $$\bar{X} \pm t\, S_{\bar{X}}$$

$$\text{where } S_{\bar{X}} = \frac{S}{\sqrt{n}}$$

One-group t-test $$t = \frac{\bar{X} - \mu}{S_{\bar{X}}}$$

$$\text{where } S_{\bar{X}} = \frac{S}{\sqrt{n}}$$

Two-group t-test

(a) when both groups have a sample size greater than 30

$$t = \frac{\bar{X}_1 - \bar{X}_2}{S_{\bar{X}_1 - \bar{X}_2}}$$

$$\text{where } S_{\bar{X}_1 - \bar{X}_2} = \sqrt{\frac{{S_1}^2}{n_1} + \frac{{S_2}^2}{n_2}}$$

and where $df = n_1 + n_2 - 2$

(b) when one or both groups have a sample size less than 30

$$t = \frac{\bar{X}_1 - \bar{X}_2}{S_{\bar{X}_1 - \bar{X}_2}}$$

$$\text{where } S_{\bar{X}_1 - \bar{X}_2} = \sqrt{\frac{(n_1 - 1){S_1}^2 + (n_2 - 1){S_2}^2}{n_1 + n_2 - 2}\left(\frac{1}{n_1} + \frac{1}{n_2}\right)}$$

and where $df = n_1 + n_2 - 2$

Correlation

$$r = \frac{\frac{1}{n-1}\sum\left(X - \bar{X}\right)\left(Y - \bar{Y}\right)}{S_x\, S_y}$$

where S_x = standard deviation of X
and where S_y = standard deviation of Y

Simple linear regression

$Y = a + bX$
where a = y-intercept and b = slope of the line

Multiple regression equation

$Y = a + b_1X_1 + b_2X_2 + b_3X_3 + \text{etc.}$
where a = y-intercept

One-way ANOVA F-test

$F = MS_b/MS_w$

ANOVA t-test

$$ANOVA\ t = \frac{\bar{X}_1 - \bar{X}_2}{s.e._{ANOVA}}$$

where $s.e._{ANOVA} = \sqrt{MS_w\left(\frac{1}{n_1} + \frac{1}{n_2}\right)}$

and where $df = n_{TOTAL} - k$
where $n_{TOTAL} = n_1 + n_2 + n_3 + \text{etc.}$
and where k = the number of groups

Appendix E: t-Table

Critical t-values needed for rejection of the null hypothesis (see Fig. E.1)

Fig. E.1 Critical t-values Needed for Rejection of the Null Hypothesis

sample size n	degrees of freedom df	critical t
10	9	2.262
11	10	2.228
12	11	2.201
13	12	2.179
14	13	2.160
15	14	2.145
16	15	2.131
17	16	2.120
18	17	2.110
19	18	2.101
20	19	2.093
21	20	2.086
22	21	2.080
23	22	2.074
24	23	2.069
25	24	2.064
26	25	2.060
27	26	2.056
28	27	2.052
29	28	2.048
30	29	2.045
31	30	2.042
32	31	2.040
33	32	2.037
34	33	2.035
35	34	2.032
36	35	2.030
37	36	2.028
38	37	2.026
39	38	2.024
40	39	2.023
infinity	infinity	1.960

Index

T.J. Quirk, S. Cummings, *Excel 2016 for Social Work Statistics*, Excel for Statistics,
DOI 10.1007/978-3-319-66221-3

Printed in Dunstable, United Kingdom

91343449R00152